Praise for
The Benjamin Franklin Diet

*"Look no further than this book to lose weight.
I highly recommend* The Benjamin Franklin Diet,
a fun and healthy way of losing weight."
—DR. DAVID ALBIN, M.D., F.A.C.S.

"The key to losing weight is diet and exercise. Benjamin Franklin, the author, inventor, scientist, and statesman, was a genius—a man before his time. So many of his life principles are followed today. Unknown to me were his writings on eating a healthy diet. His principles regarding diet are, for the most part, scientifically correct even though he wrote them without an educated background. He was a self-educated man. As a scientist and inventor, Franklin was able to utilize basic scientific principles of observation to derive the most logical conclusions.

"As a physician and surgeon for over twenty-five years I am constantly educating my patients regarding dieting. The most successful weight loss programs involve reducing one's daily intake of food and exercising. These are among the principles in *The Benjamin Franklin Diet*. The principles that impressed me the most were the simplest ones of all. You need to look no further than this book to lose weight.

"I highly recommend *The Benjamin Franklin Diet* book, a fun and healthy way of losing weight."

Dr. David Albin, M.D., a physician and surgeon for over twenty-five years, is the Medical Director for the Hernia Center of Southern California and the Pasadena Surgery Center, LLC. Certified by the American Board of General Surgery, a fellow of the American College of Surgeons, and a qualified medical examiner, Dr. Albin has authored many medical articles and ha- *b*--
to the staff of several respected hospitals.

T0273397

"*The Benjamin Franklin Diet* is a very worthwhile book offering readers approachable and delicious solutions for losing weight in a healthy way and keeping it off for life. In the midst of our nation's fat crisis, we only have to step back in time with *The Benjamin Franklin Diet* and apply the health and nutritional advice laid out by Founding Father, Benjamin Franklin.

"In our fast-food world of super-sized portions and processed junk food, this book shows us that it's not so hard to get back to basics—in fact going back to basics with wholesome, nutritious food is easier and more affordable than ever. Not only did Benjamin Franklin recommend a simple diet of natural foods, but his advice to exercise, both aerobically and with weights, has been proven to burn fat and build muscle.

"Benjamin Franklin once wrote in a letter, 'Be careful in preserving health, by due exercise and great temperance.' Wise words from a man who understood the connection between mind and body."

—SAMANTHA RAPHAEL, YOGA EXPERT

Samantha Raphael is a highly trained professional yoga instructor. She has practiced and taught yoga for more than a decade at studios, corporations and health clubs in Chicago, Illinois.

"I read the book and love it. I think even those who are gluten intolerant can stick to grains like corn and rice and older recipes and feel great.

"I have been a holistic medical doctor for many years and helped many patients with their weight and metabolism. I realized after reading this book that Benjamin Franklin was actually very correct in his principles and way ahead of his time. A gradual reduction of the stomach volume and under-eating or eating light meals is a principle I have come across in Asian cultures. There is much medical research to support eating less for longevity. The principle Franklin mentions for exercising before meals makes a lot of sense. The body is then energized and can digest, with good blood flow, the meal itself. I am fascinated to try some of the recipes myself and can see that people following the diet will be rewarded with a rich variety of recipes, a steady and maintainable weight loss, and increased energy.

"This is a wonderful book and I am happy to recommend it to people and my patients!"

—DR. HELEN K. SMITH, HOLISTIC MEDICAL DOCTOR, NEW ZEALAND

THE
BENJAMIN
FRANKLIN
DIET

Lose Weight and Live Longer with These Health Secrets from America's Founding Father

Based on the Writings of Benjamin Franklin

KELLY WRIGHT

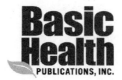

The information contained in this book is based upon the research and personal and professional experiences of the author. It is not intended as a substitute for consulting with your physician or other healthcare provider. Any attempt to diagnose and treat an illness should be done under the direction of a healthcare professional.

The publisher does not advocate the use of any particular healthcare protocol but believes the information in this book should be available to the public. The publisher and author are not responsible for any adverse effects or consequences resulting from the use of the suggestions, preparations, or procedures discussed in this book. Should the reader have any questions concerning the appropriateness of any procedures or preparation mentioned, the author and the publisher strongly suggest consulting a professional healthcare advisor.

Basic Health Publications, Inc.
28812 Top of the World Drive
Laguna Beach, CA 92651
949-715-7327 • www.basichealthpub.com

Library of Congress Cataloging-in-Publication Data
Wright, Kelly
    The Benjamin Franklin diet : lose weight and live longer with these
health secrets from America's founding father : based on the writings of
Benjamin Franklin / Kelly Wright.
        p. cm.
    Includes bibliographical references and index.
    ISBN 978-1-59120-301-8
    1. Franklin, Benjamin, 1706-1790. 2. Cooking, American. 3. Cooking, American—
History—17th century. 4. Cooking, American—History—18th century. I. Title.
    TX703.W75 2012
    641.5973—dc23

                                                            2012014243

Editor: Roberta W. Waddell
Typesetting/Book design: Gary A. Rosenberg
Cover design: Mike Stromberg

Printed in the United States of America

10   9   8   7   6   5   4   3   2   1

Contents

Important Note

Before proceeding with this book, there is something essential to be aware of concerning Benjamin Franklin (1/17/1706–4/17/1790). Take a good look at the portrait of him on the book's cover and note his slim figure, the one he had for most of his life. This is significant because the mental image of the man that pops into most people's minds is that of a kindly older person with spectacles and a paunch. And this leads to the inevitable question of how this slightly rotund man could possibly have valid diet information to impart and why anyone would ever want to take advice on eating from him, no matter how brilliant he was. The truth is, the famous Joseph Siffred Duplessis portrait of him that is firmly ensconced in people's minds is *not at all representative*. Franklin was fit and trim most of his life, up until his mid-seventies when he sat for this portrait. At that time, he was living in France and had put on extra pounds due to a combination of rich French cuisine and decreased physical activity.

Acknowledgments

Throughout my research of this book, I've met many wonderful people who shared my excitement about re-creating the diet of Founding Father Benjamin Franklin. Carly Hansen and the fantastic people at Pleasant Hill Grain believed in this book so much that they sent me two of their grain mills, as well as samplings of organic whole grains to experiment with. Thank you for your generosity.

I would like to thank my agent, Claire Gerus, for believing in this book as much as I do. I have treasured your insight and wise advice. Also, to my brilliant editor, Roberta Waddell, your enthusiasm for *The Benjamin Franklin Diet* has been as great as mine. You have a magical way with words and your suggestions and ideas made this book even better.

A big thank-you to my son, Nick Reno, and our friend Nicklas Lindskog for the sometimes brutal reviews of those early test recipes I served for dinner. You guys could have spared my feelings and said everything tasted great, but your honesty made me a better cook and the author of a better book.

Finally, I want to acknowledge my husband, Tommy Wright, my best friend and true love. Thank you for lending a few of your Ben-friendly recipes to the book and for making everything so much fun. It is a joy to have you by my side in the kitchen, and pure bliss to hold your hand as we move forward together in life.

Foreword

When I was first asked to write the foreword for a diet and weight-loss book, I have to admit, I was skeptical. I have been a registered dietitian in both the medical and fitness fields for over ten years, and I thought to myself, "Just what we need, another diet book." However, I was curious to see what advice Ben Franklin had about diet and nutrition. He did live twice as long as his peers, and let's face it, he was smart, successful, and had a few significant accomplishments in his lifetime!

The author, Kelly Wright, was struggling with her weight, and she was able to successfully lose weight by following Ben's diet guidelines, without the *pain and suffering* of most diets. She was so enthusiastic about her findings that I agreed to read her manuscript. I read it in one sitting, and found it to be an easy, healthy, sensible, and unique approach to weight loss. There are many ways to lose weight, but this collection of Benjamin Franklin's findings, theories, and recipes, is inspiring, easy to follow, and just makes sense overall.

This is not your typical diet book, and that is a primary reason why I agreed to write this foreword. It was fascinating to learn about Ben's diet principles, which I recommend you write down and review daily as a way to stay inspired and motivated. Even though I am a nutrition expert, I admit my diet is not perfect, and I do not know *everything* about nutrition. After reading this book, I even learned a few new things—it really convinced me to switch to organic products, and consume fewer animal products; yes, some dietitians do occasionally eat steak.

Much of what Benjamin Franklin preached is what I teach my patients today. In those days, consuming meat, fat, and alcohol meant you were wealthy. The way Ben ate, mostly vegetarian, with very little meat and alcohol, indicated you were poor. As we now know through research, those *wealthy*, obese, meat and alcohol consumers are today known as our heart disease, diabetes, and coronary-artery-bypass patients.

Overall, I was intrigued by the way the nutrition information was presented through Benjamin Franklin's teachings. I felt fortunate to be able to have such valuable insight and actual diet information from a brilliant man who is long gone, but will never be forgotten. Even if you don't bake your bread from scratch or cook every day, Ben's life lessons and diet principles are reason enough to read this magical book, which is *not* just another diet book.

—Lisa DeFazio, M.S., R.D.

Nutritionist and television personality Lisa DeFazio earned her Masters Degree in Nutritional Science from Cal State University in Los Angeles. She is a registered dietitian and weight management specialist certified by the American Dietetic Association. Lisa studied at the Pritkin Longevity Center and at Cedars Sinai. She was the health educator at Kaiser Permanente for eight years and the nutritional consultant on the CBS television series Big Brother. *Lisa is currently a special correspondent for Perez Hilton's celebrity website fitperez.com. She owns and operates her own weight-loss consulting business, the Diet Squad, and has been interviewed as a diet expert by* Us Weekly, STAR Magazine, *CBS, and* FOX.

How Ben Franklin Helped Me Lose Weight

*T*his may sound odd, but I'm a big fan of Benjamin Franklin. It all started when I picked up a copy of Franklin's autobiography in an airport many years ago. Believe it or not, the story of his life is a page-turner and I found myself reading it over and over again whenever I needed a lift or a little bit of inspiration in my life.

I recently celebrated my fortieth birthday. Besides a few gray hairs, I noticed that I was gaining weight faster than I used to, and that I had less energy. While I've never been obese, I was getting dangerously close to wearing plus-size clothing and my level of physical activity was almost nonexistent. The time had come for me to make some major changes in my life. But what was I to do? Like most people, I'd tried dieting and would lose the weight only to put it back on again. I didn't want to go back on a low-carbohydrate diet, but what choice did I have? I'd lost up to thirty pounds doing this in the past and it was the best solution I had.

Soon after this fortieth birthday, I put myself on a strict, low-carbohydrate diet. I lost five pounds within a couple of weeks. But as I dined on meat, cheese, fat, and artificial sweeteners, I noticed I had no energy and it seemed like the food I was eating was making me sick. *This diet can't be healthy,* I thought, but I wasn't really sure what I should be eating or how to go about achieving long-term good health. Here I was at forty years of age asking the same old question, *What am I supposed to eat?*

That's when Benjamin Franklin's autobiography came to mind. I remembered that he had written various things about diet and nutrition. So once again, I picked up the book and took notes on every reference Franklin made to food, diet, nutrition, and exercise. Then I went through letters and other documents he'd written and did the same thing. I began implementing Franklin's advice on what to eat and started to see immediate results. That was the moment I knew I'd stumbled onto something big.

Benjamin Franklin lived twice as long as the average man of his time and enjoyed good health throughout the majority of his life, which he credited to his diet. But it wasn't the typical colonial fare of red meat and ale that kept Franklin in good health—he developed his own diet, which was quite different from what everyone else was eating in eighteenth-century America. Unlike most people of the time, Franklin wasn't gorging on wild game and alcohol. He was practicing a simple diet that consisted mainly of whole grains.

A case can, in fact, be made that, besides this legendary polymath's genes and his natural brilliance, Benjamin Franklin was able to do so many things so well *because* of his exceptional style of living. It was foundational. It didn't weigh him down and, unlike many in his century, he wasn't walking around in a stupor from excessively heavy meats and fats, not to mention intemperate alcohol consumption. Clearheaded, he had the energy to be all he strove to be. His eating and exercising habits were light-years ahead of his time—he subsisted very well on a diet that, 200 years later, is scientifically recognized as a boon to good health and longevity. When he passed away at eighty-four, his lifespan was almost twice that of his contemporaries who usually died from sickness and disease in their forties or fifties, victims of the debilitating diet of the time. Think what a ripple effect there would have been if Franklin *hadn't* followed a sober diet and had been a drunk or died of disease at age forty-two like the average man. Just imagine that.

Once I had pieced together the basic principles of Franklin's diet, it was time to start developing the recipes. It wasn't long before I came to the conclusion that our food today is drastically different from the food of Colonial America. We've got fast food and processed foods that are tainted with pesticides, herbicides, chemicals, artificial sweeteners, hormones, and God only knows what else. Knowing that today's run-of-the-mill food wasn't going to cut it, I began another research project to find out exactly what foods were available in the eighteenth century and how they were prepared. Then I set out to re-create Franklin's healthy diet for today's world.

My research for *The Benjamin Franklin Diet* has been a cross-country adventure. Over the space of a recent summer, I took myself on a self-guided tour of eighteenth-century taverns, which was something like traveling back through time. I sat in real taverns in the original colonies, sampling authentic cuisine, and I haunted the dusty aisles of rare book-shops in search of long-forgotten cookbooks. Eventually I came home and put on my apron. Armed with a few kitchen utensils and a stack of colonial cookbooks written in ye olde English, I spent months in the kitchen testing authentic eighteenth-century recipes, which were more like guidelines than actual instructions. But after hundreds of test batches, I developed more than fifty authentic colonial recipes to go along with Franklin's dietary recommendations.

Throughout my research, I ate nothing but my test recipes and lost all the excess weight I'd packed on over the previous years. After a few months of following Benjamin Franklin's diet, I was as thin as I'd been in high school and had never felt better in my life. It was more than just a diet for me. I had stumbled onto a whole new way of living.

As a bonus, I discovered that each of Benjamin Franklin's recommen-dations about nutrition had been scientifically proven through contem-porary clinical research studies. Every time I came across a new reference on food, I would check it against medical studies and was able to verify that his recommendations are in alignment with today's research on healthy eating.

Besides changing my diet, I began following Franklin's exercise advice and found myself growing stronger every day. I had an incredible amount of energy, so much so that my dogs had a hard time keeping up with me on our daily walks.

Through my personal researching into *what to eat*, I found the answers in the writings of Benjamin Franklin. It is my goal to share this informa-tion and help other people get on the road to real and lasting health. The majority of Americans are overweight and unhealthy, and they don't know what they're supposed to eat. Franklin's advice solves all of these problems.

WEIGHT LOSS VS. DIET

I'd like to mention a small but important refinement concerning the words *weight loss* that are used interchangeably with *diet* throughout this book. The concept of weight loss is a contemporary construct not in the picture in Ben Franklin's time when rich people were considered the fortunate ones because their well-filled-out physiques showed they had an abundance of food. Portliness was generally associated with wealth, whereas poor people were thin because they couldn't get enough to eat—and who wanted to be poor?

The principles that Franklin espoused did not pertain to his *losing* weight. Although not from humble circumstances, he was on the thin side in childhood and his good nutritional habits—he chose not to participate in Colonial America's dreadful diet—kept him that way for most of his long life. His principles focused instead on living a simple, frugal life marked by restraint and moderation, especially regarding the too-heavy consumption of meat and alcohol by most colonists.

In this book, the term *weight loss*, a twentieth-century concept, will alternate with *diet*, except when directly referring to Franklin himself. Since current attitudes toward health frequently revolve around weight-loss principles, it is perfectly fine to call them that in the books subtitle because the book is written from today's point of view. It is not, however, fine to graft them onto Franklin's principles for his own good health, which, against the prevailing customs of his time, included exercising and his temperate, sparing diet, but not weight loss.

Poor Richard, 1733:

AN

Almanack

For the Year of Chrift

1733,

PART ONE

Ben Franklin's Lifetime Principles

Being the Firft after LEAP YEAR:

	Years
and make fince the Creation	7241
By the Account of the Eaftern Greeks	6932
By the Latin Church, when ◯ ent. ♈	5742
By the Computation of W.W.	5682
By the Roman Chronology	
By the Jewifh Rabbies	

Wherein is contained

The Lunations, Eclipfes, Judgment of the Weather, Spring Tides, Planets Motions & mutual Afpects, Sun and Moon's Rifing and Setting, Length of Days, Time of High Water, Fairs, Courts, and obfervable Days.

Fitted to the Latitude of Forty Degrees, and a Meridian of Five Hours Weft from London, but may without fenfible Error, ferve all the adjacent Places, even from Newfoundland to South-Carolina.

By RICHARD SAUNDERS, Philom.

PHILADELPHIA:

Printed and fold by B. FRANKLIN, at the New Printing-Office near the Market.

1

What You Don't Know about Ben Franklin

$\mathcal{B}$enjamin Franklin, America's most influential founding father, gained fame and honor for his achievements as an author, entrepreneur, inventor, scientist, political activist, statesman, and diplomat. Perhaps the accomplishments of his celebrated and colorful life were so monumental that we've overlooked his extensive advice on diet—quite possibly his greatest contribution to mankind.

Nearly 300 years ago, Franklin developed a revolutionary new way of eating after he discovered the secrets to a healthy diet. In an age when the life expectancy of an adult was forty-two years, Franklin not only outlived the average colonist by double, but he enjoyed good health throughout the majority of his life.

The Benjamin Franklin Diet reveals Franklin's findings as he searched for the answer to the one question that plagues everyone: *What am I supposed to eat?*

BENJAMIN FRANKLIN'S SIX PRINCIPLES OF DIET

The Benjamin Franklin Diet is based on Franklin's six principles of diet. These key precepts have been extracted from his writings and they provide the framework for a safe and delicious approach to shedding unwanted pounds—*and keeping them off for good.*

Throughout Franklin's lifetime, he wrote much about his observations and experiments on diet. After studying his advice and putting all his collective works together, several recurring themes appeared and became the basis for the six weight-loss principles. Each principle is thoroughly explained in its own chapter. The six are as follows:

1. Eat to live, don't live to eat.

2. Eat not to dullness and drink not to elevation.

3. Eat and drink no more than the body needs.

4. Eating grain brings health and vigor.

5. Remain consistent with the portions and type of food you eat.

6. There are no gains without pains.

The Ben Franklin Diet was developed using Franklin's principles, which unlock the secrets to losing weight. Following the advice outlined in this book can put you on your way to permanent weight loss and good health. And combining this advice on diet with flavorful colonial cooking make Franklin's dietary principles deliciously easy to implement.

BENJAMIN FRANKLIN'S BREAKTHROUGH DISCOVERIES

Benjamin Franklin lived an extraordinary life. But until now, little has been known about his discoveries in the field of diet and health.

As an entrepreneur, Franklin started and operated his own successful printing and publishing business, which he eventually sold for a handsome sum, allowing him to retire from business at an early age to pursue his other interests. Franklin went on to found Philadelphia's first hospital, a fire department, and the nation's first public library. As a scientist, he tamed lightning with his famous kite experiments, and invented the lightning rod, bifocal glasses, the Franklin stove, and even a musical instrument called the glass 'armonica.

While Franklin enjoyed much professional success, times in the American colonies were turbulent. The people, including Franklin, were growing tired of England's tyranny, so he turned his full attention to founding a new country where freedom could reign. He was one of the first brave souls to propose the idea of an independent American nation. At first he suggested a peaceful unification of the colonies and England. But the British rejected his proposals of peace, and he ultimately stepped to the forefront of the fight against England, becoming a key architect of the Declaration of Independence. Using his fame and influence as a scientist and statesman, Franklin took on the role of acting as America's first diplomat, and he single-handedly worked to secure the support of the French during the Revolutionary War. Franklin's success in allying the French with the revolutionaries was key to turning the ideals of a new, free nation into reality.

As one of the most celebrated men of all time, Benjamin Franklin significantly shaped the world of today. But of all the things he is remembered for, Franklin's breakthroughs in the fields of health and diet are the least known of his discoveries. To understand how Franklin came to his conclusions about diet, it's helpful to look at what eating was like in Colonial America.

FOOD IN COLONIAL TIMES

The original colonists landed on the shores of America in 1620. Although they had traveled across the Atlantic carrying the seeds for European grains and plants, it would be decades before they would successfully cultivate those crops. Instead, relying on the help of the Native Americans, the early settlers learned to plant and harvest the plentiful supply of squash, berries, corn, and other indigenous plants of the new world. As time went on, the colonists developed a taste for America's fruits, vegetables, wild game, and fish. This cornucopia of new foods, combined with crops and imports from Europe, provided a bountiful harvest for most colonial families. With 90 percent of the people involved in farming, the colonists' new world was truly a land of plenty.

A typical dinner table of the colonial period featured a variety of meats, cheeses, bread, pastries, and fruit at every sitting. Across the Atlantic in England, it was customary for the wealthy and the middle-class to eat vast quantities of meat, while root vegetables, such as potatoes and carrots, were thought of as food for animals or the extremely poor. Staying true to their English heritage, colonists dined on meat as the main course and boiled their vegetables down to a mush, if they even bothered to prepare vegetables at all.

Researchers at the American Society for Cancer Research believe that the average American colonist consumed well over 5,000 calories per day from a fatty, meat-heavy diet with few fresh vegetables. And this, in combination with large quantities of sweets, bread, cider, and rum, was a recipe for disaster.

As a young man living in the early eighteenth century, Benjamin Franklin found himself surrounded by people of ill health. His peers were dulled by alcohol, his countrymen were crippled with disease and plagues, while fevers were sweeping through the land bringing misery and death.

Franklin devoted much of his time to combating disease and improving health conditions for his fellow man, but his research into diet began accidentally when he was a teenager. While working as a printer's apprentice, Franklin's meager salary wasn't enough to afford both meat *and* books. So, being an avid reader, he opted for a more economical vegetarian diet in order to fund his one passion—reading. If his original concern was to save money, by adopting the vegetarian principles of Thomas Tryon, Franklin soon discovered that eating a diet light on meat had other benefits—it not only sharpened his mind, but also improved his comprehension when studying.

Through keen observation of his compatriots and much experimentation with his own diet, Franklin began to develop his fundamentals of healthy eating, which he expanded after studying the eating habits of indigenous people and realizing that the strongest cultures around the world lived on diets consisting primarily of whole grains. Additionally, he observed that when this type of whole-grain diet was complemented with fruits, vegetables, and small portions of meat and fat, the human body thrived. By studying the Native Americans, Franklin discovered the exact quantity of food needed to attain maximum health and optimum weight. By this point in his research, he had shed his strict vegetarian diet, but did retain its workable principles.

By isolating two key points: 1) what to eat; and 2) how much to eat,

Franklin developed his own personal diet, and this was the basis for his six principles of diet. His ideas about healthful nutrition were not only correct at the time, they are still harmonious with today's research on healthy eating. Although Franklin wasn't a medical doctor, his writings have been checked against current medical and clinical research studies and found to be in alignment with today's standards for a healthy weight.

One of Franklin's famous quotes was, *"Three good meals a day is bad living."* When he wrote this line, he wasn't advising anyone to eat fewer than three times a day. On the contrary, Franklin always ate breakfast, lunch, and dinner, and the key to his diet was eating three *light,* nourishing meals based on protein-rich whole grains. One of his most profound discoveries was just how little food the body needs. A woman in a boarding house where Franklin stayed lived entirely on a diet of gruel, a simple porridge made of whole oats. *"She was never sick,"* Franklin wrote. *"I gave it as another instance on how little is needed to support life and health."*

Being both wise and frugal with his money, Franklin adopted the old woman's routine and thereafter made his breakfast a bowl of oatmeal. As for supper, he often made an entire meal of a chunk of bread, some fish, or a handful of raisins. Discovering that light meals kept his head clear, he concluded, *"a full belly makes a dull brain."*

WHAT YOU EAT ON THE BEN FRANKLIN DIET

The Benjamin Franklin Diet, based on Franklin's timeless advice, was designed to help navigate contemporary Americans through the wide variety of food that is available today. If you choose to follow the six simple principles discovered by Franklin, you'll eat less while absorbing the maximum amount of nutrition needed to achieve and maintain your ideal weight. And don't worry. You're not going to starve to death or go hungry if you follow the guidelines laid out by Benjamin Franklin. On the contrary, you'll be full and satisfied because his revolutionary ideas and simple wisdom unlock the secrets of proper nourishment for the human body.

If you're wondering what kind of food Benjamin Franklin recommended, chances are you'll be surprised by what he said. Utilizing the wide array of colonial spices normally reserved for holiday cooking, the

Ben Franklin Diet could be compared to eating Thanksgiving or Christmas dinner every day of the week (without the miserable feeling of being overstuffed). Imagine the pleasure of losing weight as you eat fresh-baked bread, homemade butter, creamy oatmeal, rich soups, hearty stews, roasted turkey, warm gingerbread, vanilla custard, and delicious fruit pies. Read this last sentence again because *these foods are part of the Ben Franklin Diet and you are going to lose weight eating them.*

This isn't a fad or a crash diet. It's a sensible approach to losing weight in a safe, gradual manner. People who follow the Ben Franklin Diet should expect to lose a sensible one to two pounds per week.

Included in this book is a complete colonial cookbook with more than fifty authentic recipes for use on this diet. Everything is natural, there are absolutely no artificial sweeteners or chemicals used. In all ways except colonial cuisine's overdependence on meats and alcohol, the Ben Franklin Diet is true to its origins, and the food is simple and delicious. It almost sounds too good to be true, but when these foods are prepared with wholesome ingredients and eaten in proper proportions, they nourish the body and allow excess weight to fall off.

If you're thinking that dining on such seemingly decadent food will be too expensive, you should know that Franklin's fare costs a fraction of what you may already be spending on groceries. If you currently consume pre-packaged foods, microwave meals, canned soup, and convenience foods, you can expect to cut your grocery bill in half.

The illuminating advice you are about to read was discovered in the writings of Benjamin Franklin. Other pertinent information includes colonial recipes of Americans, their cooking methods, and research into their eighteenth-century foods. The recipes have been extracted from history books, journals, almanacs, colonial taverns, and rare cookbooks. They have been tested and are suitable for cooks of all skill levels, even novice.

All cultures have their own indigenous diets. You're about to discover the first one tailor-made for the American people, developed by our founding father Benjamin Franklin.

Poor Richard, 1733.

AN

Almanack

For the Year of Christ

1733,

PART TWO

Ben Franklin's Six Diet Principles

Being the First after LEAP YEAR:

And makes since the Creation | Years
By the Account of the Eastern Greeks, | 7241
By the Latin Church, when ☉ ent. ♈ | 6932
By the Computation of W.W. | 5742
By the Roman Chronology | 5682
By the Jewish Rabbies | 5494

Wherein is contained

The Lunations, Eclipses, Judgment of the Weather, Spring Tides, Planets Motions & mutual Aspects, Sun and Moon's Rising and Setting, Length of Days, Time of High Water, Fairs, Courts, and observable Days.

Fitted to the Latitude of Forty Degrees, and a Meridian of Five Hours West from *London*, but may without sensible Error, serve all the adjacent Places, even from *Newfoundland* to South-*Carolina.*

By RICHARD SAUNDERS, Philom.

PHILADELPHIA:

Printed and sold by B. FRANKLIN, at the New Printing-Office near the Market.

2

FIRST PRINCIPLE
Eat to Live, Don't Live to Eat

If Men will Feast and make Merry,
then let their Tables be spread with Philosophical Discourses.
—THOMAS TRYON, 1691

Contrary to popular myth, Benjamin Franklin was not always overweight. Evidence suggests that this founding father was trim and fit up until his mid-seventies.

According to biographer Walter Isaacson, Franklin was physically striking: almost six feet tall, he was muscular, barrel-chested, and openfaced. A portrait believed to be the earliest likeness of Franklin was painted by Boston artist Robert Feke when Franklin was forty-five. The portrait depicts him as tall, trim, and rosy-cheeked. At the time, Franklin was a successful entrepreneur and was portrayed as a prosperous Philadelphia businessman.

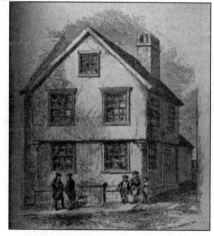

Franklin House on Milk Street, Boston.

Another portrait by James McArdell represents Franklin as a trim man in his fifties and a model of good health. The most famous paintings of Franklin, though, were created by Joseph Siffred Duplessis in the late

1700s when Franklin was living in France. At the time Franklin sat for these portraits, he was in his mid-seventies and had put on weight due to rich French cuisine and decreased physical activity. The artist painted what he saw; the chubby Benjamin Franklin we're all familiar with. But although Franklin had a generous waistline in his golden years, he was remarkably healthy throughout his life, even by today's standards.

Robert Feke's portrait of Ben Franklin.

One of Franklin's famous sayings was, *"Eat to live, and not live to eat."* As a testament to his own principle, he lived to be eighty-four years old, more than twice the life expectancy of the average man in those times. Franklin had made some remarkable discoveries about health and diet, all in a time when little was known about the human body. He avoided contracting the diseases and plagues of the day, and attributed his good health and long life to one thing—his diet.

Franklin ate plain, bland food for the most part, and he didn't allow his appetite to rule his life. In those times, less emphasis was placed on food than today when there is great importance placed on every bite eaten. Never before in history has there been such variety, with as many choices available as there are now—drive-through, fast food, Chinese takeout, sushi bars, sports bars, coffeehouses, and similar. Food has become intertwined with entertainment, making the meal the main event—a destination in itself. It's almost as though everyone has lost sight of the purpose of food, which is simply fuel for the body.

Franklin advised, *"Never eat for pleasure."* While eating can and should be a pleasurable experience, eating for pleasure alone is a one-way ticket to obesity.

To comprehend Franklin's logic about eating to live, and not living to eat involves an understanding of his humble upbringing. Benjamin Franklin was born in Boston in 1706, the fifteenth child of Josiah

Franklin, a candle- and soap-maker. Benjamin was raised in a Puritan household where the children were taught the value of hard work, discipline, and frugality.

The Puritans were educated people who ensured that their children learned to read and write at an early age so they could study the scriptures. They believed that every person should read and understand the Bible in a private way, thus forging a bond between the individual and God.

Benjamin was sent to Boston Latin School for two years, but due to financial hardship, his father was not able to keep paying the tuition. As brief as Benjamin's formal education was, however, he'd been introduced to reading and writing, which became his lifelong passion. As a child, for example, he read Bunyan's *Pilgrim's Progress* along with every other book he could get his hands on.

Benjamin's father, Josiah, was a respected man of good character who was often sought out by the townspeople for his sound advice and ability to arbitrate disputes. As a boy, Benjamin Franklin recalled frequent visits from neighbors dropping by to consult with his father. At dinnertime, the Franklin household became a place of education; a rich meeting of the minds. In a time before radios, televisions, or automobiles, the Franklin family and their frequent guests gathered to discuss the latest news, swap information, entertain each other with stories or music, and provide companionship. Virtually no attention was paid to the simple food that had been prepared without frills, for the conversation at hand was always more delicious than any dish on the table. Further, when the day's work was finished, dinner wasn't a time for discussing the food, it was a time for taking up important topics and family matters.

Of dining at his father's house, Franklin wrote: *"At his Table he lik'd to, as often as he could, [have] some sensible Friend or Neighbour, to converse with, and always took care to start some ingenious Topic for Discourse, which might tend to improve the Minds of his Children. By this means he turn'd our Attention to what was good, just and prudent in the Conduct of Life; and little or no Notice was ever taken of what related to the Victuals on the Table, whether it was well or ill drest, in or out of season, of good or bad flavour, preferable or inferior to this or that other thing of the kind."*

With conversations, and sometimes tempers, running hot at dinner,

Franklin found his total disregard of food to be a great advantage. Because he wasn't concerned with what he was eating, he never developed the finicky tastes of the upper classes.

"I was bro't up in such a perfect Inattention to those Matters as to be quite Indifferent what kind of Food was set before me; and so unobservant of it, that to this Day, if I am ask'd I can scarce tell, a few Hours after Dinner, what I din'd upon. This has been a Convenience to me in travelling, where my Companions have been sometimes very unhappy for want of a suitable Gratification of their more delicate, because better instructed, Tastes and Appetites."

As the family gathered around the dinner table, large napkins were tied around the neck and two-tined forks and knives were for the sole purpose of cutting the food. Meals were still eaten with the fingers, as silverware wouldn't come into fashion for another seventy years. Candles made of beeswax or fragrant bayberry provided dim lighting in the room, setting the scene for a typical eighteenth-century dinner at the Franklin house. The simple meals consisted of little more than a loaf of thick-crusted bread, and cornmeal mush or stew from the vegetables and grains on hand. It wasn't the food that young Franklin looked forward to every evening, it was the tantalizing conversation that was sure to take place. Franklin's utter inattention to the meals on the dinner table was the beginning of his sensible eating habits that served him well throughout his life. At an early age, he learned to appreciate good company and mentally stimulating conversation, an upbringing that taught him to hunger for knowledge, not for food.

SUMMARY

- The first step to a lifetime of healthy eating habits is to get your attention off of food and onto life.

- And always try to take Ben Franklin's advice to eat to live and not live to eat.

3

SECOND PRINCIPLE
Eat Not to Dullness and Drink Not to Elevation

If thou art dull and heavy after Meat,
it's a sign thou hast exceeded the due Measure.

—BENJAMIN FRANKLIN

Benjamin Franklin became a vegetarian at an early age, not for the love of animals, but for other reasons entirely. This chapter will take a look at his experimentation with vegetarianism and how it shaped his viewpoint on diet, eating meat, and drinking alcohol.

Benjamin Franklin's passion for reading began at an early age. During the two years he was able to attend school, Franklin developed a lifelong hunger for knowledge and learning. Because of his love for books, at the age of twelve his father sent him to work as an apprentice to his older brother James, who owned a print shop in the city. By the time Franklin was fifteen, his brother was publishing Boston's first newspaper, *The New England Courant,* which printed articles on local news, shipping schedules, and advertisements from merchants and shopkeepers.

As the newspaper was getting off the ground, young Franklin found that he didn't have enough money to pay for food and rent and still have enough left over to fund his one passion—reading. Books were expensive in the colonies and the meager salary of a printer's assistant didn't allow for such expenditures.

Despite the high price of books, however, Franklin occasionally scraped together enough money to buy a single volume. One such purchase was a cookbook by an author named Thomas Tryon, laboriously titled, *Wisdom's Dictates Including a Bill of Fare of Seventy Five Noble Dishes of Excellent Food Far Exceeding Those Made of Fish or Flesh, Which Banquet I Present to the Sons of Wisdom*, believed to be the first vegetarian cookbook ever written. Tryon advocated eating a diet entirely without meat and listed recipes to prepare meals made of grains, vegetables, and dairy products. Tryon wrote that eating *"flesh and blood"* was a depraved custom and believed that it was possible to achieve health, happiness, and long life by eating grains, plants, and dairy, including eggs.

Always looking for ways to save money, Franklin implemented Tryon's vegetarian diet and was able to save over half of the wages he earned as James's assistant. By cutting meat out of his diet, he was not only able to purchase more books, he was able to move out of his brother's house into lodgings of his own. Franklin wrote in his autobiography, *"I made my self acquainted with Tryon's Manner of preparing some of his Dishes, such as Boiling Potatoes, or Rice, making Hasty Pudding, & a few others. I presently found that I could save half what he paid me. This was an additional Fund for buying Books. But I had another Advantage in it. My Brother and the rest going from the Printing House to their Meals, I remain'd there alone, and dispatching presently my light Repast, (which often was no more than a Bisket or a Slice of Bread, a Handful of Raisins or a Tart from the Pastry Cook's, and a Glass of Water) had the rest of the Time till their Return, for Study, in which I made the greatest Progress from that Greater Clearness of Head & quicker Apprehension which usually attend Temperance in Eating and Drinking."*

During this period of Franklin's life, he learned the value of eating lightly, a discovery that served as the foundation of his lifelong dining habits. At the top of his list, Tryon recommended eating bread and oatmeal and drinking water. He said of the regimen, *"Bread and water hath the first place of all foods, and are the foundation of dry moist nourishment. Take oatmeal and make it into a gruel and put bread into it and season it with salt. This and bread and a glass of water, a man may live very well."*

Franklin believed that a diet without meat sharpened his mind and improved his comprehension. This was in alignment with the beliefs of several ancient religions and cultures following a vegetarian diet, such as the Hindus in India and some Buddhists in Asia. One of the old Hindu texts, *Mahabharata*, says that *"those who do not eat animal flesh will have good memory, long life and perfect health."* In ancient Greece, some of the great philosophers, including Socrates and Plato, believed in eating vegetarian diets.

While Franklin followed Tryon's strictly vegetarian diet for some time, he eventually began eating fish again, claiming to love hot cod that was fresh out of the frying pan. Even though he had started eating fish and fowl again, the majority of his diet consisted of whole grains. He experienced firsthand how little it took little to sustain the body, and more importantly, how eating little or no meat kept his head clear and made absorbing knowledge effortless.

Franklin continued reading and studying while he worked for his brother setting type. But he eventually grew restless with the mundane work of a printer's assistant. Although still a teenager, Franklin was ready to take on bigger challenges. He approached his brother and told him he wanted to be a writer for the paper, but James forbid it. Not willing to let his brother discourage him, Franklin assumed the pen name, *Silence Dogood*, a fictional widow who wrote critical and satirical essays about life in and current events in Boston. Franklin, a.k.a. Dogood, began sending letters to his brother's newspaper, which were carefully slipped under the door of the office late at night. James began printing the letters in his paper and the people loved them. Silence Dogood was a big hit. After many of these letters had been published, James discovered that his little brother had been writing them all along. He was angry about the hoax, and rather than giving young Franklin a job as a writer, James refused to let his brother write another word.

A short time later, Franklin ran away to Philadelphia where he found work as an apprentice to another printer. He was so skilled at his work that the Governor of Pennsylvania took notice of his talents and offered to set him up in his own business. Franklin agreed, packed his few belongings, stopped by the local bakery to stock up on loaves of gingerbread, and got on a ship to London where he was going to purchase his own printing equipment. But mid-voyage the Governor changed his mind about financing the print shop, and Franklin was left stranded and penniless in a foreign country. He had no choice but to find work in a print shop until he could earn enough money to buy his own passage back home to the colonies. It was during these trying times in London that Franklin learned some valuable lessons about temperance, frugality, and what one should and shouldn't consume in the Land of Plenty.

Sticking to his mainly vegetarian diet, Franklin was able to save his money and keep his head clear.

FRANKLIN'S EARLY LESSONS

Because the water supply in Colonial America was sometimes unsafe and polluted, especially in densely populated cities, people drank large quantities of alcohol to quench their thirst. The first settlers drank water only when necessary, and when the tea and spirits from England ran out, people began distilling their own hard alcohol from the native Indian corn, as well as alcoholic cider from apples. Excessive drinking among the colonists was common. The custom grew even more popular when farmers began cultivating crops of malt and hops. Beer, cider, and rum were the most popular drinks among the populace, much preferred over milk and water.

Most people believed that alcohol consumption was healthy and that the practice cured many common ailments. The trend of heavy drinking continued throughout the Revolutionary War and didn't taper off for many years to come.

In the late 1700s, a United States Government study showed that people over the age of fifteen consumed an annual average of thirty-four gallons of beer or cider, five gallons of distilled spirits, and one gallon of wine. But America wasn't the only place plagued by heavy alcohol consumption. The custom of drinking large quantities of alcohol was as commonplace in England as it was back in the colonies.

After the Governor of Pennsylvania reneged on the offer to set Franklin up in his own printing business and he found himself stranded in London, it became clear to him that he was surrounded by a society drowning in alcohol. He soon found employment in a print shop. Again, because his salary was small and he needed to save his money to buy passage back to the colonies, Franklin put his frugality to the test. It was during this period of his life that he found how very little he could live on.

THE WATER-AMERICAN

In the early 1700s, when Franklin worked as a typesetter in the London printing house, it was standard practice for workers to drink large quantities of cider and ale at breakfast and throughout their workday. As a means of saving money as well as keeping his mind clear, Franklin refused to drink ale as his peers did and opted for water, a decision that earned him the nickname *Water-American* among the other workers. Of this experience, Franklin wrote, *"I drank only Water; the other Workmen, near fifty in Number, were great Guzzlers of Beer. On occasion, I carried up and down Stairs a large Form of Types in each hand, when others carried but one in both Hands. They wonder'd to see from this and several Instances that the Water-American as they called me was stronger than themselves who drunk strong Beer. We had an Alehouse Boy who attended always in the House to supply the Workmen. My Companion at the Press, drank every day a Pint before Breakfast, a pint at breakfast with his Bread and Cheese; a Pint between Breakfast and Dinner; a Pint at Dinner; a Pint in the Afternoon about Six-o'clock, and another when he had done his Day's-Work. I thought it a detestable Custom. But it was necessary, he suppos'd, to drink strong Beer that he might be strong to labour."*

Not only was Franklin physically stronger than his co-workers, but his head was clearer. Franklin's sobriety paid off and he was soon promoted to dispatcher, which paid more and required less physical labor. Franklin never did mention the source of his water, but years later he wrote about the benefits of bottling water. *"You can be sure of having it good only by bottling it from a clear spring or well and in clean bottles."*

HOW LITTLE IT TAKES TO LIVE ON

In London, Franklin rented an inexpensive room in a boarding house on Duke Street from the old woman who owned the house, and he often kept her company. She was a widow who had been raised as a Protestant, but had been converted to Catholicism by her late husband. As amused as Franklin was by the little old lady who rarely ventured outdoors, he learned an important lesson about a temperate diet from her. *"Our supper was only half an Anchovy each, on a very little Strip of Bread & Butter, and half a Pint of Ale between us,"* he wrote, noting that it didn't take much food to live.

Enjoying the company of the charming young American, the widow introduced Franklin to the other boarders in the house, including an elderly maiden of seventy who lived alone in the small garret room. She too was a Roman Catholic and had once aspired to become a nun. In her younger years, she went abroad to try it out. But unfortunately, the nunnery in the foreign country she had moved to did not agree with her, so she soon returned to England. This posed a problem though... because there were no nunneries in England, she was unable to live out her dream. Instead, she vowed to live the life of a nun, with or without a nunnery to reside in. *"She had given all of her Estate to charitable Uses, reserving only Twelve Pounds a Year to live on, and out of this Sum she still gave a great deal in Charity, living her self on Watergruel only,"* Franklin wrote. *"She look'd pale, but was never sick, and I gave it as another Instance on how small an Income Life & Health may be supported."*

While Franklin was at the London printing house, he made a breakthrough discovery about the human body and how it assimilates whole grain. It all began when one of the other workers was trying to convince Franklin of the benefits of drinking beer. The worker adamantly believed that the stronger the alcohol, the more physical strength one would have. After thinking the matter over, Franklin came to a conclusion and dished out some wise advice. *"I endeavour'd to convince him that the Bodily Strength afforded by Beer could only be in proportion to the Grain or Flour of the Barley dissolved in the Water of which it was made; that there was more Flour in a Pennyworth of Bread, and therefore if he would eat that with a Pint of Water, it would give him more Strength than a Quart of Beer."*

Before the discovery of the calorie, Franklin observed that the energy from food was only as good as the proportion of grain it contained. He also noted that the human body only fully assimilates a few ounces of food per day, and if more than the required amount was consumed, the body turned it to waste. Franklin's theory was to get the maximum amount of nutrition from food without overloading the body with excess matter to process. His observation about eating grain itself rather than drinking beer made from grain is an example of taking nutrition directly from the source for maximum benefit.

Although his stay in London was brief, Franklin made a lasting impression on the other workers in the print shop. *"From my Example a great Part of them left their muddling Breakfast of Beer & Bread & Cheese, finding they could with me be supply'd from a neighbouring House with a large Porringer of hot Water-gruel, sprinkled with Pepper, crumb'd with Bread, & a Bit of Butter in it, for the price of a Pint of Beer, viz, three halfpence. This was a more comfortable as well as cheaper Breakfast, & kept their Heads clearer."*

By using his keen power of observation, Franklin came to some wise conclusions about diet while overseas. He revisited and reinforced his earlier discovery that light meals kept his head clear, had no ill-effects on the body, and improved comprehension when studying, and then wrote the famous line, *"a full belly makes a dull brain."* Franklin had long-since adopted the old nun's routine of eating hot-water gruel (oatmeal) for breakfast, and despite the great wealth he would acquire later in life, he always remained temperate with food and alcohol. Unlike his peers in the upper class, Franklin chose simple, wholesome foods and wrote about his habit of eating a mere slice of bread or some fish or a handful of raisins for a meal.

SUMMARY

- Eating a light diet keeps the mind clear and improves comprehension.

- Less meat and more grains is not only frugal, but better for the body and mind.

- The proportion of grain assimilated by the body is only as good as its source.

- The body only processes a few ounces of food per day and turns the excess to waste.

4

THIRD PRINCIPLE
Eat and Drink No More Than the Body Needs

To lengthen thy life, lessen thy meals.
—BENJAMIN FRANKLIN

$\mathcal{U}$pon his return to Philadelphia, Franklin worked as an assistant to another printer. Within a short time, Franklin went into business for himself. Frugally watching every penny, he worked well into the night at his print shop. By carting his own supplies through the streets in a wheelbarrow and living temperately, his business began to prosper. Franklin married Deborah Reed, a woman as frugal as he was. Being wise entrepreneurs, the Franklins opened a small general store to generate more income. Despite the wealth they were accumulating from their shop and printing business, Franklin never forgot the lessons he'd learned about sensible eating and frugal living. In his autobiography, he described his standard breakfast as bread and a little milk served in a cheap earthen bowl and eaten with a pewter spoon.

As Thomas Tryon's vegetarian cookbook advocated, *"Let your Food be simple, and Drinks innocent, and learn of Wisdom and Experience how to prepare them aright."* A simple, nutritious diet is the key to a lifetime of good health. The idea is to get your attention off of food and onto sustaining the body. This may sound difficult, even distasteful, but when your health and vigor return, you may never eat the same again. While much of the diet is plain, the food is wholesome and certainly isn't without taste. More importantly, the food is what the human body needs to obtain maximum health. The Ben Franklin Diet is about eating to live, and not living to eat.

Franklin wrote, *"I went home in the evening, purchased a twopenny loaf at the baker's, and with the water from the pump made my supper; I then wrapped myself up in a green-coat, and laid down on the floor and slept till morning, when, on another loaf and a mug of water, I made my breakfast. From this regimen, I feel no inconvenience whatsoever."*

While a slice of bread for supper may not seem like enough to survive on, a dense piece of bread in Colonial America was quite different than white bread today. A slice of brown bread in Franklin's day made a simple and satisfying meal. Made with whole-grain flour, buttermilk, butter, and unrefined sugar or molasses, this heavy, whole-grain bread provided plenty of carbohydrates and protein to properly nourish the body. Franklin noted that eating meat made him feel dull and tired, and he believed that food should give people energy and make them feel light.

Contrary to popular myth, whole grains or cereals provide almost half the protein in the world's diet, not meat. Frances Moore Lappé, author of the bestselling book *Diet for a Small Planet,* discovered that combinations of proper proportions of non-meat foods can produce high-grade protein nutrition that is equivalent to, or better than, protein from meat sources. Lappé wrote that the average American eats almost twice the protein the body can use and concluded that if meat, fish, and poultry were eliminated from the diet, people could still get their recommended daily allowance of protein, about 58 grams, from other protein-rich foods, such as grains, plants, and dairy. Additionally, a plant-centered diet rich in whole grains, legumes, fresh fruits, and vegetables provides excellent fiber content. The low fiber content found in the typical, highly processed American diet has been linked to intestinal blockage, appendicitis, and cancer. Lappé's conclusions are in precise alignment with Franklin's beliefs about a proper, plant-based diet that is light on, or entirely free of, meat.

In 1786, Franklin wrote a letter of advice to his friend Catherine Shipley about the quantity of food needed to achieve optimum health, noting that active adults needed more food than inactive adults, and that intake should be adjusted accordingly. *"Observe however, that Quantities of Food and Exercise are relative things; those who move much may, and indeed ought to, eat more; those who use little Exercise should eat little. In general, Mankind, since the improvement of Cookery, eats about twice as much as Nature requires. Suppers are not bad if we have not din'd, but restless Nights naturally follow hearty Suppers after full Dinners."*

HOW MUCH FOOD DOES THE BODY NEED?

The human stomach needs about one pint of food to fill it. Consider how much food that actually is. Have you ever gone to a restaurant and eaten bread and butter before the meal? Did you feel full and satisfied before your food arrived twenty minutes later? You get the idea. It doesn't take much to fill the stomach.

Nutrition expert Robyn Flipse, R.D., says that stomach size expands and contracts according to the amount of food you eat. If you practice eating small meals and don't overfill the stomach, the capacity it can hold will be less and you won't feel hungry as often. But just as the stomach shrinks, it also expands when we overeat consistently, which could happen by eating large dinners or meals, even just once a day. Occasional overeating won't expand the stomach, but some experts believe that overeating at meals for two to four weeks can change the shape of the stomach and require more food to fill it at a sitting.

Dr. David Albin, M.D., agrees with Benjamin Franklin's advice—to keep meals small and in the one-pint range. He believes that light meals have no negative effects on the body and can help improve comprehension. "It is a proven scientific fact that if you eat less, your stomach will shrink and it will take less to satiate your appetite," says Dr. Albin. "You are going to lose weight and without being hungry."

Dr. Matovu, a gastroenterologist at Kibuli Hospital in Kampala, Uganda, says it is a medical fact that people can decrease their stomach size by changing their diet, and that it takes less than one month to do so by eating small, evenly spaced meals. Dr. Lawrence Cheskin, M.D., head of the Weight Management Center at Johns Hopkins School of Medicine, recommends eating three moderate meals a day at regularly scheduled intervals. In the beginning, your appetite may be bigger than your stomach, so practice temperance as the size of your stomach decreases. *"To lengthen thy life, lessen thy meals,"* Franklin advised.

Never skip meals and *save up* for a big meal later. Eat at regular intervals and never consume more than one pint per sitting. You'll find that if you keep your meals in the one-pint range, you won't be hungry all the time as your stomach capacity adjusts to a more temperate eating style.

SIX OUNCES OF GRAIN SHALL SUSTAIN

Franklin observed early on that it didn't take much food to live on. After adopting the breakfast routine of the old woman in the boarding house, he knew that a bowl of oatmeal eaten with butter or a piece of bread with milk would suffice for breakfast, and he followed this simple eating regimen for much of his life. In his autobiography he wrote, *". . . my Breakfast was a long time Bread and Milk, (no Tea) and I ate it out of a twopenny earthen Porringer with a Pewter Spoon."*

Living on a diet consisting primarily of whole grains, Franklin concluded that six ounces of uncooked ground meal a day was enough to sustain the average man. As a large man himself, he suffered no ill effects from this diet and was in good health.

The average adult stomach will hold about a pint of food or liquid. It can expand to hold up to four pints of food or liquid at a time, but one pint is all that is needed to create the sensation of feeling full. Franklin wrote a letter in 1785 about the benefits of Indian corn, or maize, ground into a meal after observing how the Indians of North America survived on a small portions of it quite well. *"An Indian will travel far, and subsist long on a small Bag of it, taking only 6 or 8 Ounces of it per day, mix'd with Water."* Six to eight ounces of uncooked grain will expand to about eight cups, or four pints. In the 1756 edition of *Poor Richard*, Franklin wrote of eating rice and how six ounces of uncooked brown rice would be sufficient food for one person per day.

HOW MUCH CAN I EAT ON THE BEN FRANKLIN DIET?

You are allotted up to eight cups (four pints total) of food per day on the diet, which include three one-pint meals, plus one pint of snacks. Snacks can be eaten throughout the day, but never immediately preceding or following a regular meal. Only eat snacks if you are truly hungry. If you're full and satisfied on three pints of food per day, don't bother eating snacks at all.

Although the diet is based on consuming four pints of food per day, some people's bodies will require slightly less, while others will require slightly more. One way to discover your ideal amount of food is to make a loose fist and compare it to the size of a one-cup measuring cup. An average adult hand is about the size of one cup. If your fist is considerably larger than one cup, you may need more food, and if it's smaller, you probably need less food.

When you first start the diet, begin with four pints (eight cups) of food per day and see how you feel when you eat slightly more or less. Also, if you have a very active lifestyle and are burning lots of calories, you may need more food; if you have little activity in your day, your body may require less. Monitor how you feel when you eat certain proportions. The key is to discover the proportion that is perfect to nourish your body and provide the proper amount of energy to fit your lifestyle.

After a week or two of the Ben Franklin Diet, you will discover the correct amount of food to sustain your body. Once that amount is known, use moderation when eating, and stick to it.

In the *Farmer's Almanac* of 1756, Franklin published recipes for making different meals out of ground grains, noting that it only takes a minimal amount of food to sustain a man for a day. *"That six Ounces of Meal should sustain a Man a Day is not unlikely, when it is considered, that it is almost all capable of being converted into Nourishment; that Nature does not absolutely require so much neat Addition daily to the Substance of the Body, the therefore Full-feeders, by frequent Evacuations, discharge a great Part of their common Food not completely digested; but where so small a Quantity is admitted, the Discharges will be less frequent, and the Food moving slower through the Intestines, and being retained longer within them is almost wholly assimilated."*

While six to eight ounces of dry grain doesn't sound like much, when the whole grains are cooked, they can double or triple in weight and volume, depending on what type they are. Combine the six to eight ounces of whole grains with some leafy green vegetables, a portion of turkey, chicken, or fish, finished off later with some fresh, seasonal fruit, and you're eating pretty well. For instance, an ounce of whole-wheat flour is equivalent to one slice of dense bread, and two ounces of steel-cut oats is equivalent to two cups of cooked oatmeal. The idea is to nourish the body without overeating, which can make you feel sluggish and dull. By eating less and fully assimilating your food, your mind will be clearer, your body lighter, and you'll be on your way to the proverbial health, wealth, and wisdom.

Refer to Recipes, Part Three, Chapter 11 for an index of grains. You'll begin with an allowance of six cups of cooked grains as a daily minimum. As you choose your meals from the menu, you'll be able to see the grain value and customize it to suit your tastes. That grain can be cooked rice, oatmeal, whole-grain bread, whole-grain soup, whole-grain pasta, or one of the many other choices found in this book. If you find that six cups of grain is too little or too much, all you have to do is add or delete some of it from your diet until you find the quantity that is right for your body. You don't have to be perfect, and you don't have to count calories. The idea is to discover what your body needs and what works for you personally. With the grain-value charts and portions already calculated next to every recipe, all you have to do is pick out what you want and start eating.

FRANKLIN'S GUIDELINES TO DETERMINE HOW MUCH TO EAT

Writing as Poor Richard, Franklin's 1742 edition of the *Farmer's Almanac* outlined his rules to moderate how much food and drink is needed to achieve optimum health. Begin with six cups of cooked grains, along with vegetables and small portions of easily digestible meat, and small portions of seasonal fruit. From this foundation, you can develop a diet that is suited to your exact needs. Look at Franklin's guidelines below and see the sample meal plan section of this book.

Poor Richard's Rules to Find a Fit Measure of Meat and Drink

- If thou eatest so much as makes thee unfit for Study, or other Business, thou exceeded the due measure.

- If thou art dull and heavy after Meat, it's a sign thou hast exceeded the due Measure; for Meat and Drink ought to refresh the Body, and make it cheerful, and not to dull and oppress it.

- If thou findest these ill Symptoms, consider whether too much Meat, or too much Drink occasions it, or both, and abate by little and little, till thou findest the Inconveniency removed.

- Keep out of Sight of Feasts and Banquets as much as may be; for 'tis more difficult to refrain good Cheer, when it's present, than from the Desire of it when it is away; the like you may observe in the Objects of all the other Senses.

- If a Man casually exceeds, let him fast the next Meal, and all may be well again, provided it not be done too often; as if he exceed at Dinner, let him refrain from a Supper.

- A temperate diet Frees from Diseases; such are seldom ill, but if they are surprised with Sickness, they bear it better and recover sooner; for most Distempers have their Original from Repletion.

- Use now and then a little Exercise a quarter of an Hour before Meals, as to swing a Weight, or swing your Arms about with a small Weight in each Hand; to leap, or the like, for that stirs the Muscles of the Breast.

- A temperate diet Arms the Body against all external Accidents; so that they are not so easily hurt by Heat, Cold or Labour; if they at any time should be prejudiced, they are more easily cured, either of Wounds, Discolorations or Bruises.

- But when malignant Fevers are rife in the Country or City where thou dwelst, 'tis advisable to eat and drink more freely, by Way of Prevention; for those are Diseases that are not caused by Repletion, and seldom attach Full-feeders.

- A sober diet makes a Man die without Pain; it maintains the Senses in Vigour; it mitigates the Violence of Passions and Affections. It preserves the Memory, it helps Understanding, it allays the Heat of Lust; it brings a Man to a Consideration of his latter End; it makes the Body a fit Tabernacle for the Lord to dwell in; which makes us happy in this World, end eternally happy in the World to come, through Jesus Christ our Lord and Saviour.

SUMMARY

- The stomach needs no more than one pint of food per meal to fill it.

- Habitual, light eating reduces the capacity of the stomach.

- Six cups of cooked grain per day is all that is needed to sustain the average adult.

- Practice temperance and avoid overeating.

5

FOURTH PRINCIPLE
Eating Grain
Brings Health and Vigor

All may reflect how light, how well they were,
when plain and simple was their cheerful Fare.
—BENJAMIN FRANKLIN

*T*hroughout history, some of the strongest cultures in the world ate diets of whole grains. Rations for soldiers of the Roman Army consisted of wheat, which was ground into meal to make porridge and bread. This grain-based diet was supplemented with other available foods, such as pork, fish, chicken, vegetables, and fruit. But the soldier's daily ration of whole grains was the key.

The foundation of the Ben Franklin Diet is built on whole grains. It is recommended on this diet that 75 percent of your daily food intake consist of complex carbohydrates, mainly made of whole grains. This is in alignment with recommendations from the World Health Organization and the Food and Agricultural Organization, which jointly recommend that national dietary guidelines set a goal of getting up to 75 percent of total energy from complex carbohydrates.

In the *Farmer's Almanac* of 1756, Franklin observed and wrote about the health benefits of eating whole grains. *"The Poor in many countries live mostly on some sort of grain Powder diluted with boiling Water, and often with cold Water, particularly the Natives of America, who in their Huntings, or in the long Marches they sometimes make to meet and fight their Enemies, have nothing to subsist on but a little Meal made of Indian Corn; and that*

35

after having subsisted for many Weeks of Months solely on this Diet, they are not only healthful and vigorous, but the Wounds they receive in Battle are cured with surprising Facility."

Franklin observed that the Indians were strong and healthy, as were other grain-eating cultures, such as the Chinese, East Indians, and Romans, whose traditional diets still center around whole grains and who use meat as a garnish rather than a main course.

The traditional Asian diet consists of up to 75 percent whole grains, mainly from rice. Besides helping the body maintain a healthy weight, diets rich in whole grains have been found to prevent heart disease and cancer. Today in China, the death rate from heart disease is seven times lower than it is in America and the colon-cancer rate among the Chinese is three times lower than that of Americans.

Author and nutritionist Adelle Davis wrote about the advantages of eating whole-grain breads and cereals, as proven during World War I, when food shortages caused the Danish government to forbid the milling and refining of grains. Because the people were eating only whole grains, nutrition in Denmark improved so greatly that during the war years, the national death rate fell by 34 percent. This remarkable statistic was due to a sharp decrease in cancer, diabetes, heart disease, high blood pressure, and kidney disease. Much the same improvement occurred in England during and after World War II, when grains were only slightly milled.

The average American today eats almost twice the amount of protein the body can process, so the leftover protein turns to waste. By cutting down on protein derived from meat sources and eating whole grains, it's easy to create a fully digestible meal with little waste.

While proteins, carbohydrates, fats, and even calories were unknown in Franklin's time, his advice on nutrition aligned with today's recommendations to eat a diet of complex carbohydrates in combination with small portions of protein and even fats, as for example, his advice to eat a bowl of oatmeal with a small amount of butter or a piece of whole-grain bread with an anchovy. Little did he know how this combination of complex carbohydrates with protein and fat works beneficially to slow down the process of digestion and create a full feeling in the stomach that lasts for a long time.

A brief look at complex carbohydrates and simple carbohydrates will show how this carbohydrate/protein/fat mechanism works.

Complex carbohydrates, such as whole-grain bread, brown rice, oatmeal, and many vegetables that are digested slowly by the body do no not result in large spikes in insulin levels. Think of complex carbohydrates as time-release capsules of energy.

On the other hand, simple carbohydrates, such as refined sugar, white-flour products, and some fruits, can be thought of as direct injections of energy into the bloodstream. This is because they digest and absorb quickly, and this results in large, sudden bursts of insulin that lead to energy crashes afterward. Once your energy crashes, you're more susceptible to cravings, which can only be satisfied by consuming more simple carbohydrates. It's a vicious circle.

If you're trying to lose weight, you want to slow down your rate of digestion and ensure that your insulin levels are steady. By knocking out the simple carbohydrates and replacing them with complex carbohydrates, you can slow the body's speed of digestion and make the rate of insulin production steady. And when this rate is steady, the body has no need to convert excess energy into fat for storage.

Because fats and proteins digest even more slowly than complex carbohydrates, adding small amounts of them to each meal, as Franklin did, markedly slows down the body's process of carbohydrate digestion. As a result, energy from the carbohydrates is released at slow, steady levels, providing the body with energy and making weight loss possible.

Vegetables are a source of complex carbohydrates that should be included as part of your daily intake. The Centers for Disease Control and Prevention (CDC) recommends substituting fresh vegetables for higher calorie foods as a way to add volume and fiber to your meals. As an example, they recommend swapping two ounces of meat on a sandwich with the same amount of lettuce, tomatoes, and onions—in other words, eat the same number of ounces while consuming fewer calories.

Tip. As a way to gauge how healthy your meals are, the CDC recommends looking at your dinner plate before you eat. Whole grains, vegetables, and fruits should make up the largest portion of the plate. If they do not, replace some of the meat, cheese, or simple carbohydrates, such as white pasta or white rice, with vegetables to reduce the total calories of the meal without reducing the size of the meal.

WHOLE GRAINS

The most common source of complex carbohydrates is whole grain.

Whole grains, and foods made from them, consist of the entire grain seed or kernel. The kernel is made of three parts; bran, germ, and endosperm.

The Three Parts of Grain

1. **Bran,** or fiber: The exterior outer protective layer of the kernel. Rich in B vitamins and a good source of fiber.

2. **Germ:** The interior part of the seed. A source of minerals, protein, vitamins B and E, and oils.

3. **Endosperm:** The large interior part of the kernel protected by the bran. A source of some proteins and mainly starch.

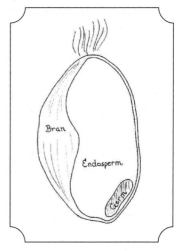

A whole-grain kernel and its parts.

Once grains are crushed into meal or flour, whole grains consist of all three parts with nothing removed. As one example, a kernel of corn, the seed, contains all three parts, and when it is ground, it becomes whole-grain cornmeal.

Refined grains, on the other hand, have had one or more of these parts removed. In the grain-refining process, most of the bran and some of the germ is removed, resulting in the loss of dietary fiber, vitamins, minerals, and other nutrients. White rice is a good example of a refined grain where some or all of the bran and germ have been removed, and the remaining endosperm is bleached to whiten it. Although refined grain has a longer shelf life than whole grains, without the bran and germ, the rice loses much of its fiber, fats, oils, minerals, antioxidants, and vitamins.

Examples of whole grains include wheat, oats, corn, millet, barley, rice, rye, and sorghum. In the Colonial American diet, grains consisted mainly of oats, wheat, rye, barley, corn, and rice. Although the dishes on the tables got fancier and forks came into fashion, eighteenth-century food remained much the same as seventeenth-century food in Colonial America. Corn and other grains were a mainstay of the colonial diet and were ground and eaten whole, not refined as they are today.

To compare: A slice of whole-grain wheat bread has ninety calories and four grams of protein while a slice of today's white bread has eighty calories and two grams of protein. You can pretty much count on the nutritional value of refined breads having about half the amount of protein and nutrients of breads made with whole grains. Whole grains are rich in magnesium, potassium, folic acid, antioxidants, and protein-rich oils. Additionally, whole grains are an excellent source of various B vitamins, including niacin, riboflavin, and thiamin. These vitamins give the body energy and are an essential part of the body's nutritional needs.

The best way to ensure that you're buying a 100-percent whole-grain product is to carefully read the label on the packaging. Labeling on breads and cereals can be confusing and many products called *whole grain* are in fact, not. Food companies often use misleading wording, such as *multigrain, stone ground,* or *seven grain* on a product that is made with refined flour and other ingredients. The rule is, *the very first ingredient* on any such food product should be a recognizable whole grain, such as *100 percent whole-wheat flour,* or *oats.* Don't be fooled into eating anything less than a whole-grain product because of tricky advertising. Look for breads that are dense and heavy and have visible additions such as oats, barley, seeds, or coarse pieces of whole grain. The more intact the grain is, the slower the digestion will be.

Benjamin Franklin recognized the health benefits of whole grains based on his personal observations. He experienced a clear head, energy, and good health and attributed this to his diet.

Scientists are now discovering that Franklin's theories and conclusions about nutrition were correct. Researchers at Wake Forest University

School of Medicine found that people who ate diets high in whole-grain foods had a significant reduction in the risk of heart disease and strokes. Evidence was also found that eating whole grains protects against diabetes, chronic illnesses, high blood pressure, and obesity.

Currently, only 8 percent of Americans consume three or more servings of whole-grain foods per day, and 42 percent of adults eat no whole-grain foods at all. Combine that with the massive consumption of processed foods, fast food, and inactive lifestyles, and it's easy to see why nearly two-thirds of the American population is overweight, with one third falling into the obese category.

By changing to a simple diet based around delicious whole grains, health and proper weight can be restored and maintained.

Common Complex Carbohydrates

Grains and Vegetables. Artichokes, asparagus, barley, beans, bran, broccoli, brown rice, buckwheat, bulgur, celery, corn, cornmeal, cucumber, eggplant, leafy green vegetables, lentils, millet, oats, onions, pasta, peas, potatoes, quinoa, rye, tomatoes, whole-wheat bread, whole-wheat crackers, whole-wheat pasta, wild rice, zucchini

Fruits. Apples, blueberries, melon, peaches, pears, plums, pumpkin, raspberries, strawberries, watermelon

Common Simple (Refined) Carbohydrates

Any product made with corn syrup or high-fructose corn syrup, baked goods made with white flour, bread and pasta made with white flour, candy, fruit juices, soft drinks, sugar, white rice

Common Proteins

Beef, cheese, chicken, eggs, milk, nuts, pork, salmon, tuna, turkey, yogurt

THE AMERICAN FOOD SUPPLY HAS CHANGED

Most eighteenth-century families in America lived on a plot of land and farmed. For those who lived in the cities of the day, whole grains, fruits, and vegetables were readily available at markets. In summer there were blackberries, blueberries, huckleberries, and wild strawberries that were often sweetened with sugar, molasses, or honey. There were apples, beans, corn, herbs, onions, pumpkins, and an abundance of fish and wild game year round. The key to Franklin's healthy eating habits was knowing what to eat and in what proportions.

Today's Americans live in a land brimming with an endless array of unhealthy food. The meat supply is tainted with antibiotics, growth hormones, and food colorings. Many of the commercially produced dairy products come from cows that have been treated with rBGH, a growth hormone that has been linked to an increase of breast and prostate cancer.

There is a vast difference between the dairy products, wild game, and meat of colonial times and the foods available today. Even though colonial beef and pork was natural and organic, Franklin still preferred fish and fowl over red meat and felt sluggish and ill when he overindulged on it. In one account, Franklin tracked his weekly diet and noted feeling ill after several days of dining out and eating heavy meals, including beef, mutton, and pork. After taking a night off from eating out, he fasted through his supper and found that he felt better. Franklin was no purist when it came to food, but he did develop, and stick to, a simple, sensible diet, which served him well throughout his life. He occasionally ate red meat, drank a glass of wine or a pint of ale, and even dined on dolphin for breakfast while traveling overseas. But he kept his meat consumption light and ate it as a garnish rather than the main course.

Unless you grow your own grain, fruits, and vegetables, or buy organically grown foods, eating modern-day produce and grain products can be a dangerous undertaking. In colonial times, fruits, vegetables, and grains were grown on family farms using no fertilizers, pesticides, or chemicals. Food was the way nature intended it. Today, more than 99 percent of the farmland in America is exposed to toxic agricultural herbicides and pesticides that wind up in the food you eat. Not only do these chemicals get into the food, but they are transferred through meat from animals that have been fed toxic crops.

Over the last decade, genetically modified organisms (GMOs) have entered the mainstream marketplace. GMOs are the result of a laboratory process in which genes from one species are spliced into another to obtain a desired trait or characteristic. An example of a GMO food is a strawberry or a tomato injected with the genes of an Arctic fish to create a frost-resistant plant species. Another common type of GMO crop includes plants that have had herbicides and insecticides *built in* to the genes of the seeds, meaning that every time consumers bite into these foods, they are ingesting toxins.

GMO corn, cotton, soy, and other commercially grown crops are readily available on the shelves of our supermarkets and with absolutely no warning to unsuspecting consumers. For example, if your cereal was made with GMO corn, nowhere on the packaging would you be notified of it. Additionally, when these GMO products are used as ingredients in other products, such as GMO wheat in a pasta product, there will be no warning on the label. Because GMO crops have only been around for a little over a decade, the long-term effects on human health is unknown.

Various studies in animals that have eaten GMO crops have shown potentially pre-cancerous cell growth, damaged immune systems, smaller brains, livers, and testicles, and higher death rates.

The only way to avoid ingesting these untested and potentially unsafe plant, meat, and dairy products is to grow food yourself or buy organic food from the health food store or farmer's market.

Note: The integrity of organic fields is being compromised by migrating GMO seeds that, to add insult to injury, are patented. This means that the organic farmers whose fields are the unintended recipients of these unwelcome seeds are also in danger of being sued for using the seeds without payment to the patent holder. Talk about a catch-22. This is becoming a serious enough problem for the organic farmers that they are banding together to push for relief and protection from governmental powers to help them maintain the integrity of their produce against the vagaries of the wind blowing unwelcome GMO seeds their way.

SUMMARY

- Some of the healthiest civilizations in the world lived on a diet based in whole grains.

- Your daily food allowance should be 75-percent complex carbohydrates, mainly in the form of whole grains. This translates into about three pints, or six cups of cooked whole grains and some fresh vegetables and fruit per day. The remainder of your daily intake should be a combination of small amounts of dairy, small amounts of protein, and a little fat. You can get your daily grains by eating oatmeal, rice, or other cooked grains, or by eating whole-grain bread or other foods made mainly with whole-grain flour.

- Combining complex carbohydrates with small amounts of protein and fat beneficially slows down the body's digestion process.

- Eat whole, natural grains instead of refined grains to obtain maximum health.

- Eat organic food to give your body the maximum amount of vitamins, minerals, and nutrition. If possible, never skimp here. Eat only the best food available, even if it costs more.

6

FIFTH PRINCIPLE

Remain Consistent with the Portions and Types of Food You Eat

Eat for necessity, not pleasure.

—BENJAMIN FRANKLIN

WHAT IS TEMPERANCE?

The word *temperance* means to habitually moderate any indulgence of the appetites or the passions. Temperance is the ability to exhibit self-control and restraint. When it comes to what is eaten, remaining consistent with proper proportions of food is the key to losing weight and keeping it off for life.

For Americans today, it is important to develop temperance in eating habits. In a world of contradicting messages and advertisements from the food industry that provide a constant source of temptation, everyone is bombarded with advertisements for fast food, restaurants, commercially produced food products, and convenience foods that their manufacturers promote. Driving through neighborhoods, you can see billboards for fried chicken and key lime pie and the latest flavor of milk shake looming above you on every street corner. Television and radio broadcasts promise culinary delight at every commercial break if you'll just buy their products. There are cookbook stores, cooking magazines, and entire TV channels dedicated to food and cooking. Food is everywhere and the manufacturers all want one thing—to sell their products and turn a profit.

In Colonial America, taverns and merchants didn't advertise their food. People weren't constantly invited to sample one of these or one of those, or try this new food product, or dish, or restaurant. As colonists rode their horses into the village, there were no billboards promoting "Miss Ada's Hot Water Gruel." The age of advertising wouldn't begin until the following century.

The next time you're driving to work, observe how many different advertisements for food you see along the way. Count the billboards and the signs for restaurants and grocery stores. You'll be amazed by the number of advertisements you count. But more important, you'll learn to spot and ignore the messages from a food industry that isn't concerned about your health and well-being.

Although there were no advertisements for food in Colonial America, there was another type of temptation that did present itself: banquets and feasts. A typical colonial banquet featured a wide variety of meats, cheese, bread, pastry, desserts, and sugared fruits, as well as ale, cider, punch, and spirits. Franklin advised to not only be temperate, but to avoid these feasts if possible. *"Keep out of Sight of Feasts and Banquets as much as may be; for 'tis more difficult to refrain good Cheer, when it's present, than from the Desire of it when it is away; the like you may observe in the Objects of all the other Senses."*

While you might not attend banquets on a regular basis, beware of all-you-can-eat buffets and potlucks where the temptation to overeat exists. If you have to attend a banquet or potluck dinner, walk through it first to see what choices are available before you load up your plate.

THE DIFFERENCE BETWEEN
AN EMPTY STOMACH AND HUNGER

As you start the Ben Franklin Diet, you need to understand the difference between the sensations of an empty stomach and actual hunger. Most people are used to the feeling of a full stomach, and when it's empty, they tend to fill it up again. Once the stomach has processed the food, the meal moves into the intestines to be digested, but just because the stomach is empty doesn't mean it needs more food right away. This is a feeling you need to know and recognize. The feeling of hunger is different. It is the sensation of a growling, idle stomach with nothing to do and nothing to process. When the stomach growls and gurgles, it's sending a message that it's ready for you to send it more food to be processed. About two hours after the stomach is empty, it produces hormones that stimulate nerves to send a message to the brain. The brain tells the muscles in the digestive system to contract, which results in a growling or rumbling sound. If you're used to eating large portions, be aware that when you start consuming fewer calories and smaller portions, your stomach may growl between meals. You'll need to ignore that growling for the first week or two until your stomach adjusts to processing less food.

There will be times when you'll be tempted to indulge in various foods outside the sensible diet you've adopted. When these urges seem to be taking over your self-control, stop and ask yourself if you really are hungry. If you find yourself tempted to eat something just to fill your empty stomach, drink a glass of water instead, or have a light snack and, above all, practice temperance until your stomach lets you know it's time for your next meal. As Franklin advised, *"'Tis easier to suppress the first desire than to satisfy all that follow it."* If your stomach is growling before mealtime to let you know it's hungry, so what? It's perfectly natural. This is where practicing temperance comes into use. As Franklin wrote, *"Hunger is the best pickle."*

HOW TO CUT BACK ON SODAS, TEA, COFFEE, ALCOHOL, AND SWEET DRINKS

Franklin's drink of choice was water, although he sometimes drank tea, coffee, ale, and wine in moderation. Today, in contrast, people consume not only large quantities of tea and coffee, but also sodas, fruit juices, and energy drinks.

While researching *The Benjamin Franklin Diet,* I wanted to know what obese people were consuming that was causing their weight problem. In an effort to discover the answer, I spent two entire days in a grocery store, observing what was in the shopping carts of obese people. In this observational study, I found that the carts of obese shoppers all had the same two items in common—white bread and fruit juice. Combine fruit juices, especially ones sweetened with high-fructose corn syrup, with the empty calories of refined white bread and you have a surefire guarantee of weight gain. It is, in any case, far better for your health to eat a piece of raw fruit than to drink fruit juice. When you eat the whole fruit, you're getting the vitamins, water, and fiber while consuming fewer calories.

If you feel you're drinking too much caffeine, soda, fruit juice, or other types of drinks besides water, Franklin offered advice to cut back on these items, not only for good health, but also to practice frugality.

"If you are now a Drinker of Punch, Wine or Tea, twice a Day; for the ensuing Year drink them but once a Day. If you now drink them but once a Day, do it but every other Day. If you do it now but once a Week, reduce the Practice to once a Fortnight. And if you do not exceed in Quantity as you lessen the Times, half your Expence in these Articles will be saved."

Franklin's method of cutting back on alcohol was this: *"When you incline to drink Rum, fill the Glass half with Water."* This sound advice on watering down rum works wonderfully with other drinks you want to cut down on, including juice, coffee, tea, and soda.

What to Do if You've Overindulged

Okay, so you started the Ben Franklin Diet and you blew it. You went out to lunch with your co-workers at the office and stuffed yourself with heavy, fatty foods and sweets and now you don't feel so great. This happens to everyone, and it certainly happened to Franklin. His advice on handling overeating was to have a short fasting period to get the body back on track. *"If a Man casually exceeds, let him fast the next Meal, and all may be well again, provided it not be done too often; as if he exceed at Dinner, let him refrain from a Supper."*

In other words, if you overate at lunch, skip your evening meal to let your body balance out.

BREAKING A LIFETIME OF BAD HABITS

No one is perfect, especially when it comes to eating properly and taking care of the body. Is there a way to reduce or eliminate bad habits and replace them with good habits? Franklin thought so, and in his autobiography he wrote about his own method of self-improvement.

Franklin conceived what he called a *"bold and arduous project"* to achieve moral perfection. He had read what other contemporary authors considered moral virtues and had found them limited, so he came up with his own list of thirteen virtues and a method to adopt them, calling it *The Art of Virtue.* While the aim of Franklin's undertaking was to achieve moral perfection, he soon discovered that perfection was impossible. But through his self-improvement exercises, he learned much about himself and was able to overcome many of his faults.

Franklin took up one of his thirteen virtues every week and kept daily notes on his progress toward implementing them into his life.

"My intention being to acquire Habitude of all these Virtues, I judg'd it would be well not to distract my Attention by attempting the whole at once, but to fix it on one of them at a time, and when I should be Master of that, then to proceed to another, and so on till I should have gone thro' the thirteen . . . And like him who having a Garden to weed . . . does not attempt to eradicate all the bad Herbs at once, which would exceed his Reach and Strength, but works on one of the Beds at a time." Repeating the entire list of virtues every thirteen weeks, Franklin kept at it and did this exercise four times a year. Little by little, he found that many of his bad habits and flaws fell away.

Here is Benjamin Franklin's list of thirteen virtues.

1. **Temperance.** Eat not to Dullness, Drink not to elevation.

2. **Silence.** Speak not but what may benefit others or yourself. Avoid trifling Conversation.

3. **Order.** Let all your Things have their Places. Let each Part of your Business have its Time.

4. **Resolution.** Resolve to perform what you ought. Perform without fail what you resolve.

5. **Frugality.** Make no Expence but to do good to others or yourself: i.e., Waste nothing.

6. **Industry.** Lose no time. Be always employ'd in something useful. Cut off all unnecessary Actions.

7. **Sincerity.** Use no hurtful Deceit.

8. **Justice.** Wrong none, by doing Injuries or omitting the Benefits that are your Duty.

9. **Moderation.** Avoid Extremes. Forbear resenting Injuries so much as you think they deserve.

10. **Cleanliness.** Tolerate no Uncleanness on Body, Cloaths or Habitation.

11. **Tranquility.** Be not disturbed at Trifles, or at Accidents common or unavoidable.

12. **Chastity.** Rarely use Venery but for Health or Offspring; Never to Dullness, Weakness, or the Injury of your own or another's Peace or Reputation.

13. **Humility.** Imitate Jesus or Socrates.

Try this exercise of Franklin's to improve your life. Take up one virtue each week beginning with Temperance and keep a diary of your daily progress. Once you've cycled through the virtues, start with the first again. As Franklin wrote, *"I was surpriz'd to find myself so much fuller of Faults than I had imagined, but I had the Satisfaction of seeing them diminish."*

FRANKLIN'S ART OF VIRTUE

WEEK 1: TEMPERANCE

Monday	Tuesday	Wednesday	Thursday	Friday	Saturday	Sunday

WEEK 2: SILENCE

Monday	Tuesday	Wednesday	Thursday	Friday	Saturday	Sunday

WEEK 3: ORDER

Monday	Tuesday	Wednesday	Thursday	Friday	Saturday	Sunday

WEEK 4: RESOLUTION

Monday	Tuesday	Wednesday	Thursday	Friday	Saturday	Sunday

WEEK 5: FRUGALITY

Monday	Tuesday	Wednesday	Thursday	Friday	Saturday	Sunday

WEEK 6: INDUSTRY

Monday	Tuesday	Wednesday	Thursday	Friday	Saturday	Sunday

WEEK 7: SINCERITY

Monday	Tuesday	Wednesday	Thursday	Friday	Saturday	Sunday

WEEK 8: JUSTICE

Monday	Tuesday	Wednesday	Thursday	Friday	Saturday	Sunday

WEEK 9: MODERATION

Monday	Tuesday	Wednesday	Thursday	Friday	Saturday	Sunday

WEEK 10: CLEANLINESS

Monday	Tuesday	Wednesday	Thursday	Friday	Saturday	Sunday

WEEK 11: TRANQUILITY

Monday	Tuesday	Wednesday	Thursday	Friday	Saturday	Sunday

WEEK 12: CHASTITY

Monday	Tuesday	Wednesday	Thursday	Friday	Saturday	Sunday

WEEK 13: HUMILITY

Monday	Tuesday	Wednesday	Thursday	Friday	Saturday	Sunday

SUMMARY

- Practice temperance and remain consistent with the amount of food you consume.

- Stop and think before you eat, and look at whether you're really hungry or your stomach is empty. If you're in doubt, drink a glass of water and see how you feel.

- If you've overeaten, fast through the next meal.

- Try Franklin's exercise of adopting a new virtue every week.

7

SIXTH PRINCIPLE
There Are No Gains without Pains

Be careful in preserving health,
by due exercise and great temperance.
—BENJAMIN FRANKLIN

*I*n Colonial America, the majority of the population worked from dawn to dusk. Those who weren't farming were involved in other work requiring physical labor, including carpentry, tanning, milling, and blacksmithing. The men worked while the women stayed at home. It was women's responsibility to care for the children, cook, clean, sew, and take care of the household. The average colonial woman was very busy and on average gave birth to nine children. Although Colonial Americans consumed 5,000 calories a day, they burned off a good deal of them with their active lifestyles.

Today, the average American consumes 2,700 calories a day and is far less active than his/her colonial ancestors. Two-thirds of Americans are overweight or obese and 300,000 adult deaths every year in the United States are attributed to unhealthy dietary habits and inactive lifestyles. But there's good news. Researchers at the American Institute for Cancer Research say it's never too early or too late to start making healthy changes in eating habits. By transitioning to a diet that features a variety of vegetables, whole grains, fruits, and reduced portions of meat, the risk for cancer and other health problems associated with obesity are greatly reduced.

FRANKLIN'S SECRET FOR LONGEVITY

Benjamin Franklin lived to be an active eighty-four-year-old in a time
when the life expectancy of the average American was around forty. Only
a small percentage of people, including Franklin, lived to see their
seventies and eighties. So what did he do differently? As discussed, the
primary reason he lived twice as long as the average Colonial American
was the temperate way he ate, shunning the unhealthy eating customs of
his time.

FRANKLIN'S OTHER SECRET FOR LONGEVITY—
EXERCISE

Besides his superb eating habits, Franklin's other secret to long life was
exercise. In a letter to a relative, he wrote, *"The resolution you have taken
to use more exercise is extremely proper, and I hope you will steadily perform
it. It is of the greatest importance to prevent diseases."*

Exercise is a vitally important part of achieving optimum health and
happiness. Franklin found that moderate exercise *before* meals improved
his digestion, promoted sound sleep, and put him in a cheerful mood.
*"To this End it is in the first place necessary to be careful in preserving Health,
by due Exercise and great Temperance; for in Sickness the Imagination is dis-
turb'd; and disagreeable, sometimes terrible, Ideas are apt to present themselves.
Exercise should precede Meals, not immediately follow them; the first promotes,
the latter obstructs Digestion. If after Exercise we feed sparingly, the Digestion
will be easy and good, the Body lightsome, the Temper cheerful, and all the
Animal Functions perform'd agreeably. Sleep when it follows, will be natural
and undisturb'd."*

Franklin recommended light, moderate exercise fifteen minutes *before*
eating a meal. While most exercise programs will tell you to exercise after
you eat, a look at the human body will show you what it's designed for.
Exercising before meals is more in line with the body's natural makeup.
If you were a farmer, would you eat your meal and then go out and harvest
your vegetables? Of course not. This is out of sequence. You would first

have to harvest the crop before you could eat it. Hunger is the motivation for procuring food. Ancient peoples would hunt first and eat afterward, just as all mammals do. As an example, if you were to go out in the wild, you would expend your energy finding food and shelter. You would only eat *after* you had found a source of food.

Exercising before meals is in line with man's natural makeup. Dr. David Albin says, "Benjamin Franklin found that moderate exercise before meals improved digestion, promoted sound sleep, and put one in a cheerful mood. Following his principles of exercising before each meal for just fifteen minutes would add forty-five minutes of exercise to your day. Most Americans are lucky if they exercise twenty minutes three times a week."

Dr. Morrison's Miracle Guide to Pain-Free Health and Longevity strongly advises resting after a meal, never exercising. Dr. Morrison wrote, "The fact is that after eating, a person ought to rest, take it easy, never become active. Observe what the animals do. They play and romp *before* they eat. After their meal they curl up and nap. It is bad for you to do otherwise. After consuming a meal, the blood is needed in the organs for digestion. It's the fuel the digestive apparatus needs for cooking down the meal and reducing it to the normal end-products of digestion. When you walk after a meal you use the muscles of locomotion, and *they* also need blood for this. So what happens is that the muscles of walking pull some of the needed blood away from the *digesting* organs. My research has shown beyond any peradventure of doubt that activity following food consumption makes for digestive problems. It is physiologically wrong. My advice is to allow the blood to be in the digestive organs after eating. There it is needed for thorough digestion of what you've consumed."

An article on the website *MuscleandFitness.com* recommends working out *before* breakfast four to six days per week when the body is in its optimal fat-burning mode. This advice aligns with Franklin's recommendations about when to exercise. *"Use now and then a little Exercise a quarter of an Hour before Meals, as to swing a Weight, or swing your Arms about with a small Weight in each Hand; to leap, or the like, for that stirs the Muscles of the Breast."*

Leaping

Try leaping around the house or the kitchen for fifteen minutes and you'll find that, as silly as it sounds (and looks), leaping is quite invigorating and really gets the heart pumping like no other form of physical activity. Start off with small leaps from one foot to the other, using your arms to increase your lift. You may leap side-to-side, switching from one leg to the other, or leap forward, alternating your leaping leg. Leaping exercises the legs, arms, and torso all at once, providing an excellent workout.

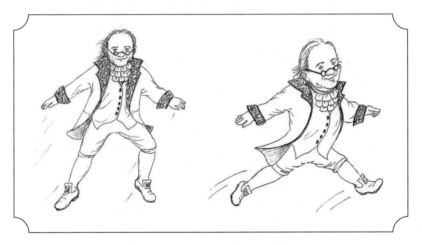

Figure 7.1. Various versions of the Franklin leap.

"O Lazy-bones! Dost thou think God would have given thee arms and legs, if he had not design'd thou should'st use them."

—BENJAMIN FRANKLIN, *POOR RICHARD'S ALMANACK*

If leaping around the house isn't your cup of tea, or if you're physically unable to leap, you may start off by lunging. You can also take a short, brisk walk before your meals to help aid digestion and burn off calories.

Benjamin Franklin found the best exercise is that which warms up the body quickly and raises the pulse. *"In considering the different kinds of exercise, I have thought that the quantum of each is to be judged of, not by time or by distance, but by the degree of warmth it produces in the body: Thus when*

I observe if I am cold when I get into a carriage in the morning, I may ride all day without being warmed by it, that if on horse back my feet are cold, I may ride some hours before they become warm; but if I am ever so cold on foot, I cannot walk an hour briskly, without glowing from head to foot by the quickened circulation."

Franklin also recommended climbing stairs as exercise. Of stair climbing he said, *"There is more exercise in walking one mile up and down stairs than in five on a level floor. The two latter exercises may be had within doors, when the weather discourages going abroad; and the last may be had when one is pinched for time, as containing a great quantity of exercise in a handful of minutes.*

Climbing stairs is a great way to get in shape, especially if the weather outdoors is unpleasant. A study in Finland found that people who climbed twenty-five flights of stairs a day lost a significant amount of weight over the course of just three months. In fact, if you were to climb just four flights of stairs a day instead of riding the elevator and changed nothing else in your life, you'd burn enough excess calories to lose twelve pounds over the course of a year.

Franklin also recommended lifting weights as a good way to raise the pulse and create warmth in the body. *"The dumb bell is another exercise of the latter compendious kind; by the use of it I have in forty swings quickened my pulse from 60 to 100 beats in a minute, counted by a second watch; and I suppose the warmth generally increases with quickness of pulse."*

In a pamphlet entitled "Proposals Relating to the Education of Youth in Pennsylvania," Franklin advised, *"Students should diet together plainly, temperately, and frugally,"* and *"be frequently exercised in running, leaping, wrestling, and swimming."*

Whatever exercise you choose, do something, and always exercise before your meals, not after. Franklin wrote, *"If your situation in life is a sedentary one, your amusements, your recreation at least, should be active."* If you aren't able to get out and walk, sweep the floors, rake leaves, or do some weeding in the garden. Walk up and down the stairs, or get out and hand-wash your car. Participate in activities that provide a good range of motion for your body.

Franklin was also fond of swimming and had studied the 1696 book

The Art of Swimming by Melchisédech Thévenot, one of the first books on the subject. The book popularized the breaststroke and was widely read during the eighteenth century.

Franklin wrote, *"I stripped and leaped into the river, and swam from near Chelsea to Blackfriars, performing on the way many feats of activity, both upon and underwater. I had from a child been ever delighted with this exercise, had studied and practiced Thevenot's motions and positions, added some of my own, aiming at the graceful and easy as well as the useful."*

Assuming you eat three times a day, exercising just fifteen minutes before each meal adds forty-five minutes of exercise to your day. Make these forty-five minutes a minimum and work toward increasing your physical activity to an hour a day.

Stop Kidding Yourself and Get Active

Everyone has heard the phrase *no pain, no gain*. As contemporary as it sounds, it was Ben Franklin who coined these famous words back in the eighteenth century when he wrote, *"There are no gains without pains."*

Exercise is essential to your health, and you must make time for it every day. Forty-five minutes of moderate exercise broken up into fifteen-minute intervals before meals is the minimum amount an adult needs every day. Exercise is not always easy and, yes, sometimes it can be painful. Just remember Franklin's famous words as you sweat it out and know that you're losing fat and gaining a healthier body. Eventually your sore muscles and pain will diminish as you grow stronger.

In Franklin's old age, he admitted that he failed to follow his own advice on getting daily exercise. In 1780, he wrote a humorous letter to himself, called *Dialogue between Franklin and the Gout*. He wrote, *"Let us examine your course of life,"* the Gout said. *"When the mornings are long and you have plenty of time to go out for a walk, what do you do? Instead of getting up an appetite for breakfast by salutary exercise you amuse yourself with books, pamphlets, and newspapers, most of which are not worth the trouble. Yet you eat an abundant breakfast . . . Immediately afterwards you sit down to write at your desk or talk with people who come to you on business. This lasts til an hour after noon, without any kind of bodily exercise . . . But what do you do after dinner? Instead of walking in the beautiful gardens of friends with whom you have dined, like a man of sense, you settle down at the chess board and there you stay for two or three hours . . . Wrapped in speculations of this wretched game, you destroy your constitution . . . Flatter yourself no longer that half an hour's airing in your carriage deserves the name of exercise. Providence has appointed few to roll in carriages, while he has given to all a pair of legs, which are machines infinitely more commodious and serviceable. Be grateful, then, and make proper use of yours . . . Remember how often you have promised yourself to walk tomorrow morning in the Bois de Boulogne, in the garden at La Muette, or in your own, and then have not kept your word; alleging sometimes that it was too cold, at other times too warm, too windy, too damp, or too something else; when in truth it was too much nothing which hindered you but too much laziness. You know Mr. Brillion's gardens and how good they are for walking; you know the fine flight of a hundred and fifty steps which lead from the terrace down to the lawn. You have been in the habit of visiting this amiable family twice a week in the afternoon. A maxim you yourself invented says that a man may have as much exercise in going a mile up and down stairs as in walking ten on level ground. What an opportunity for you to take exercise in both these ways! . . . What have you done? You have sat on the terrace, praised the fine view, and looked at the beauties of the gardens below; but you have never stirred a step to descend and walk about in them. On the contrary, you call for tea and the chess board . . . And then, instead of walking home, which would stir you up a little, you take your carriage . . . "*

"What would you have me do with my carriage?" Franklin asked.

Gout replied, *"Burn it if you like . . . or, if that proposal does not suit you, I have another. Observe the poor peasants who till the soil in the vineyards and fields about the villages of Passay, Auteuil, Chaillot, etc. Every day you may find among these good creatures four or five old women and old men, bent and perhaps crippled by the weight of years and by labour too hard and unrelieved, who after a long, fatiguing day have to walk a mile or two to their cottages. Order your coachman to pick them up and take them home. That will be a good deed, and good for your soul! And if at the same time, after your visit, you return on foot, that will be good for your body."*

"Ah! How tiresome you are," Franklin cried. "Oh! Oh! For heaven's sake *leave me! And I promise faithfully that from now on I shall play no more chess but shall take daily exercise and live temperately."*

"I know you too well," said Gout. *"You promise beautifully; but, after a few months of good health, you will go back to your old habits; your fine promises will be forgotten like the forms of last year's clouds."*

After suffering from a six-week spell of gout, Benjamin Franklin began to heed his own advice on exercise again. In a letter to John Adams dated November 20, 1782, Franklin wrote, *"I walk a league every day in my chamber. I walk quickly and for an hour, I make a point of religion of it."*

SUMMARY

- Incorporate a daily exercise routine into your life.

- Exercise moderately *before* meals, not after.

- Begin with forty-five minutes of exercise daily, broken into three, fifteen-minute intervals.

8

Franklin's Magic Formula for Success

In the Affair of so much Importance to you,
wherein you ask my Advice,
I cannot want for sufficient Premises,
advise you what to determine,
but if you please I will tell you how.
—BENJAMIN FRANKLIN

*T*his chapter is about one of the most important choices you will ever have to make—changing your diet. Choosing to adopt a healthy diet and lifestyle is a major decision. It isn't always going to be easy, yet these changes are rewarded with a lifetime of good health. The benefits of good health can't be enjoyed, however, unless you decide to make positive changes and act upon them. No one else can eat or exercise for you, just as no one else can breathe for you. Going from a lifetime of unhealthy eating habits to a healthy, temperate lifestyle is a major turning point.

What decision could be more important than to make permanent, positive changes in your diet? If you are still undecided about getting on the road to optimum health, the following exercise will help you make a decision that is best for you.

You might have heard about the famous Benjamin Franklin *Pros and Cons Formula.* This was an actual formula that Franklin used when he was faced with difficult decisions, and you can use it to come to a decision on even the toughest problem.

Read the following formula carefully. Then apply it to the subject of changing your diet. Be sure to have a piece of paper and pen handy to write down your ideas for or against the decision. The result will be a rational decision based on your own arguments.

BENJAMIN FRANKLIN'S
PROS AND CONS FORMULA

In the Affair of so much Importance to you, wherein you ask my Advice, I cannot want for sufficient Premises, advise you what to determine, but if you please I will tell you how. When these difficult cases occur, they are difficult chiefly because while we have them under Consideration all the Reasons pro and con are not present to the Mind at the same time; but sometimes one Set present themselves, and at other times another, the first being out of Sight. Hence the various Purposes or Inclinations that alternatively prevail, and the Uncertainty that perplexes us.

To get over this, my Way is to divide half a Sheet of Paper by a Line into two Columns, writing over the one Pro, and over the other Con. Then during three or four Days Consideration I put down under the different Heads short Hints of the different Motives that at different Times occur to me for or against the Measure. When I have thus got them all together in one View, I endeavor to estimate their respective Weights; and where I find two, one on each side, that seem equal, I strike them both out: If I find a Reason pro to some two Reasons con, I strike out the three. If I judge some two Reasons con equal to some three Reasons pro, I strike out the five; and thus proceeding I find at length where the Balance lies; and if after a Day or two of farther Consideration nothing new that is of Importance occurs on either side, I come to a Determination accordingly.

And tho' the Weight of Reasons cannot be taken with the Precision of Algebraic Quantities, yet when each is considered separately and comparatively, and the whole lies before me, I think I can judge better, and am less likely to make a rash Step; and in fact I have found great Advantage from this kind of Equation in what may be called Moral or Prudential Algebra.

Wishing sincerely that you may determine for the best, I am ever, my dear Friend, Yours most affectionately. Benjamin Franklin

WORKSHEET FOR PROS AND CONS FORMULA

Pros	Cons

It was Benjamin Franklin who famously said, *"An ounce of prevention is worth a pound of cure."* He believed in taking precautions to avoid problems later, and as an accomplished chess player, he was always a few moves ahead in the game.

POOR RICHARD'S ALMANACK

In 1733, Franklin began publishing *Poor Richard's Almanack.* In addition to providing him with a handsome income, the small publication provided a platform for Franklin to share his discoveries and dish out advice to the public. Almanacs of the era were printed annually and included weather reports, recipes, predictions, and homilies. Franklin published his almanac under the guise of a man named Richard Saunders, a.k.a. Poor Richard, an ordinary man who needed money to take care of his nagging wife. Many of the famous phrases associated with Franklin, such as, "a penny saved is a penny earned" came from his fictitious character, Poor Richard.

Benjamin Franklin's Rules of Health and Long Life

Franklin lived a celebrated life and offered some wise advice on how to stick around for a long time. Franklin's 1742 edition of *Poor Richard's Almanack* (published annually from 1732 to 1758) outlined his personal rules to achieve health and long life. These rules apply today just as they did in Franklin's time.

1. Eat and Drink such an exact Quantity as the Constitution of the Body allows of, in reference to the Services of the Mind.

2. They that study much, ought not to eat so much as those that work hard, their Digestion being not so good.

3. The exact Quantity and Quality being found out, is to be kept constantly.

4. Excess in all other Things whatever, as well as in Meat and Drink, is also to be avoided.

5. Youth, Age and Sick require a different Quantity.

6. And so do those of contrary complexions, for that which is too much for a flegmatick man, is not sufficient for a cholerick.

7. The Measure of Food ought to be (as much as possibly may be) exactly proportionable to the Quality and Condition of the Stomach, because the Stomach digests it.

8. That Quantity that is sufficient, the Stomach can perfectly concoct and digest, and it sufficeth the due Nourishment of the Body.

9. A greater Quantity of some things may be eaten than of others, some being of lighter Digestion than others.

10. The Difficulty lies in finding out an exact Measure; but eat for Necessity, not Pleasure, for Lust knows not where Necessity ends.

11. Wouldst thou enjoy a long Life, a healthy Body, and a vigorous Mind, and be acquainted also with the wonderful works of God? Labour in the first place to bring thy Appetite into Subjection to Reason.

Although Franklin was prosperous, he continued living simply and remained temperate with his diet. By the time he was in his early forties, he was in perfect health; this in an age when forty-two was the average life expectancy. Franklin's lifelong fascination with nutrition had paid off and his conclusions about health and diet had been correct. He'd outlived the average man and was still going strong.

In the *Poor Richard Improved* of 1756, Franklin wrote about Lewis Cornaro, the author of *Benefits of a Sober Life*. Cornaro attributed his good health and long life of 120 years to a temperate diet.

Franklin wrote, *"He says, to the fortieth Year of his Age, he was continually perplex'd with Variety of Infirmities; at last he grew so careful of his Diet, that in one Year, he was almost freed from all his Diseases. He continued thus temperate all the rest of his life, sound, cheerful and vegete, and was so entire and perfect in his Strength at Fourscore Years, as to be able to walk, ride, hunt and perform every Office of Life as well as in his Youth. At length, he died in his Chair, with very little Pain or Sickness, all his Senses being entire to the last, tho' in the 120th Year of his Age."*

Beneath Franklin's introduction to Cornaro was the following poem.

Mark, what Blessings flow
From Frugal temperate meals; 'tis they bestow
That prime of Blessings, HEALTH. All will confess
That various Meats the Stomach much oppress.
All may reflect how light, how well they were,
When plain and simple was their cheerful Fare.
Who down to Sleep from a short Supper lies,
Can to the next Day's Business cheerful rise,
Or jovially indulge, when the round Year
Brings back the festal Day to better Cheer
Or when his wasted strength he would restore
When Years approach, and Age's feeble Hour
A softer Treatment claim. But if in Prime
Of Youth and Health, you take, before your Time,
The Luxuries of Life, where is their Aid
When Age and Sickness shall your Strength invade.

"Cornaro, among other Advantage arising from Temperance, mentions this as a material one, that a Man by outliving his Competitors, arrives at higher Dignities, and more profitable Employments, and by keeping his Mind clear, his Body in Health, improves his Knowledge and Abilities, and can execute those Employments with greater Reputation. He might have added, that by living long, a Man long enjoys the Reputation and Fame he may have acquired. Aristotle was much more famous after his Death than during his Life; but Newton, who lived to the Age of 85, had been 60 Years a distinguish'd Philosopher, and many Years before he dy'd was universally esteem'd and admir'd. If Praise be, as Plato said, the sweetest Kind of Music, Newton long enjoy'd a Concert of that Music."

SUMMARY

- The decision to change your life is within you. No one can do it for you.

- Use the *Pros and Cons* formula to make good decisions in life.

- Light eating, temperance, and exercise contribute to a long and healthy life.

- Never eat for pleasure.

- Live an active life and live and enjoy the fruits of your labor.

9

Discover Your Passion in Life

Seest thou a man diligent in his calling,
he shall stand before kings.

—BENJAMIN FRANKLIN

You may be wondering what finding your passion in life has to do with the Ben Franklin Diet and the answer is, absolutely everything. As Franklin famously said, *"Eat to live, don't live to eat."*

If you often find yourself obsessing about your food or your weight, there's a good chance you're not living your dream life. By finding your passion and going after it, your whole outlook on life will change. You'll go from focusing inward and being critical of yourself to focusing your attention on the world out there and on what you want as you work to turn your dreams into reality.

Life isn't about food or exercise or dieting. Life is about curiosity and creating and living. Have you ever been so interested in something that you forgot to eat? If you are operating and living on that level, there's no time to worry about the little things. The idea of finding your passion in life is to expand outside your head and get so excited about your goals that you're 100 percent focused on making your dreams come true.

Benjamin Franklin found that when men had nothing to do, they began to find fault with small things, such as their food. *"On the idle Days they were mutinous and quarrelsome, finding fault with their Pork & Bread*

and in continual ill-humour: which put me in mind of a Sea-Captain whose
Rule is was to keep his Men constantly at Work; and when his Mate once told
him that they had done every thing, and there was nothing farther to employ
them about; O, says he, make them scour the Anchor."

We've all been there. When there's nothing to do and life seems dull
and purposeless, we tend to find fault in little things—our weight, for
example. Franklin's remedy for this was to get in action and keep busy.
He advised, *"Be Industrious. Lose no Time. Be always employ'd in something*
useful. Cut off all unnecessary actions."

But what should you do with your life? How do you go about finding
your true calling? How do you find that passion for living that occupies
your mind continually? To the question that plagues us all, *what should*
I do with my life? the great philosopher Aristotle discovered the answer:
"Where your talents and the needs of the world cross, lies your calling."

Benjamin Franklin is an excellent example of a man who found success
by following his calling in life. At age ten, he was put to work in his
father's candle-making business. Disliking this work, he studied Latin
and read books every chance he got. Reading and writing were his passions in life. When his father recognized this, he sent Benjamin to
apprentice as a printer for his older brother, for the printing business was
as close to books as his father could get him. Franklin continued to feed
his passion for reading, studying, and writing throughout his entire life.
In his autobiography he wrote, *"My circumstances, however, grew easier*
daily. My original habits of frugality continuing, and my father having,
among his instructions to me when a boy, frequently repeated a proverb of
Solomon, 'Seest thou a man diligent in his calling, he shall stand before kings,
he shall not stand before men,' I thence considered industry as a means of
obtaining wealth and distinction which encouraged me—though I did not
think that I should ever literally stand before kings, which, however, has since
happened; for I have stood before five, and even had the honor of sitting down
with one, the King of Denmark, to dinner." Franklin also wrote, *"Let every*
one ascertain his special business and calling, and then stick to it."

What is your calling in life? What is your greatest love? The quote by
Aristotle is worth reading again, for it offers the secret to discovering

your passion in life. *"Where your talents and the needs of the world cross, lies your calling."*

AN EXERCISE TO HELP YOU FIND YOUR CALLING:

Write down what you would be doing with your life if you could do *anything* you wanted. What do you dream about doing? What kinds of things do you like to do in your spare time? What are you really passionate about? What are your talents?

Now, write down all of the ways that the world could benefit from *your dreams and talents* and keep focusing on these until you realize a way to match up your dreams with the needs of the world.

SUMMARY

• Find your passion in life and seek a way to make this your life's work.

• Always work toward the goals you've set and never waste a moment.

10

Following the Rules—
Most of the Time

GETTING STARTED ON THE BEN FRANKLIN DIET

I hope you have decided to try the Ben Franklin Diet because, if you have, a life of health and happiness lies before you. To obtain maximum health benefits from the diet plan, it is recommended that you prepare your own meals. If you're not set up to bake and cook a week's worth of meals and you want to get started today, you can purchase the basics at your local health food store or farmer's market. (*See* the Quick Start shopping list at the end of this chapter.)

SIMPLE FOOD AND COLONIAL COOKERY

The food on the Ben Franklin Diet is simple, yet delicious. The idea is not to provide an endless array of culinary possibilities; it is to provide guidelines for simple, rustic food that you can remain constant with. As Franklin once said, *"Many Dishes, many Diseases."* Once you get the idea of what to eat and precisely how much food your body needs, you are encouraged to explore the fascinating world of Colonial American cooking. There are many cookbooks available on the subject, some of which are listed in References in back. Additionally, the cookbook that first inspired Benjamin Franklin to eat light, Thomas Tryon's *A Bill of Fare, Seventy Five Noble Dishes of Excellent Food,* can be found in the Appendix.

In the mid-to-late 1700s, the art of cooking had improved and imports from around the world were available in the colonies. The first cookbooks were arriving from England, and in 1742, the first cookbook of the American Colonies, *The Compleat Housewife or, Accomplish'd Gentlewoman's Companion,* by Eliza Smith, was published. From the time that the first settlers landed on Plymouth Rock in 1620, American cooking had been evolving as housewives combined old-world recipes with indigenous Indian foods. The result was a new national cuisine with influences of English, German, Dutch, Scottish, and Irish cooking. Despite the improvements and variety in food, Franklin still preferred simple fare, believing that improvements in cooking led to unnecessary overeating. He wrote, *"Mankind, since the improvement of Cookery, eats about twice as much as Nature requires."*

The recipes in this book are made with wholesome ingredients and are designed to provide proper nourishment for the body. Colonial cooking was simple, as are the foods on the Ben Franklin Diet. If you want to achieve the maximum benefits of this diet, you will need to prepare your own food, a small price to pay for a lifetime of health and happiness.

The colonial recipes in this book have been updated for convenient use in today's world, yet the wholesome ingredients that produce delicious and nutritious meals remain the same. If you're unfamiliar with the kitchen, don't let cooking intimidate you. The instructions have been simplified and tested, and are virtually foolproof.

ORGANIC AND LOCALLY GROWN FOOD

The ingredients for the recipes of the Ben Franklin Diet will cost a fraction of what you're likely spending on food right now. Invest your money wisely and buy only whole grains and organic ingredients at your local health food store or farmer's market.

While organic vegetables, fruits, grains, and other ingredients may cost a few pennies more, it's important to purchase the best food available. When you buy from a local farmer's market, you're getting fresh, just-picked produce. Fruits and vegetables at farmers' markets are usually sold within twenty-four hours of being harvested, unlike produce at grocery stores, which may have been in transit for a week or two before reaching the shelves of the store. The flavor of locally grown, fresh food will be at its peak because it hasn't been sitting in a warehouse or in a processing plant losing vital nutrients.

By shopping at a farmer's market, you'll also be able to meet the growers and ensure that they don't use harmful chemicals and pesticides. Don't skimp here. Buy only the best food.

QUICK-START SHOPPING LIST

If you're eager to start the Ben Franklin Diet right now, but aren't set up to grind grains, bake bread, and make butter, here's a shopping list to get you though the first week.

Quick-Start Shopping List for the Ben Franklin Diet

I loaf 100-percent whole-grain bread (wheat, rye, oatmeal, or multigrain)

Organic butter (salted or unsalted)

I box 100-percent rolled oats or steel cut oats

$1/2$ gallon organic whole milk

Fresh, in-season vegetables (enough for 1–2 cups per day)

Fresh, in-season fruit (enough for I cup per day)

Organic popcorn (for snacks)

Organic nuts—your choice (enough for $1/4$ cup per day as snacks throughout the week)

Cheese for snacks (cheddar, mozzarella, Swiss, or any kind except processed American)

I box of whole-grain crackers, such as Rye Krisp, Wasa, or Heart to Heart Whole-grain Crackers (Kashi)

Organic raw sugar (this sugar is golden looking and the crystals are large)

I bag brown organic rice (Lundberg from CA is a superior brand)

Organic chicken or turkey breasts, or sliced organic turkey (enough for three or four sandwiches)

Fresh fish (your choice—buy enough for 1–2 servings), or buy canned tuna or salmon for sandwiches

I head of leafy green lettuce or organic spinach for salads and sandwiches

Benjamin Franklin Meal-Replacement Energy Bars

I recommend that, in addition to the above shopping list, you purchase the ingredients for this recipe (*see* recipe in Chapter 12) and make a batch to eat throughout the week. These delicious bars are great for meals on the go. They are packed with complex carbohydrates and protein that have been perfectly balanced and specifically designed for use on the Ben Franklin Diet. It only takes one hour to prep and bake a batch of a dozen. The bars taste great and eating them can accelerate weight loss.

SCHEDULE A COOKING DAY

In Colonial America, baking and cooking was done once a week in most households. On baking days, the bread dough was made first. The oven was fired up and as the oven temperature climbed, the bread loaves were set on the hearth to rise. The loaves then went into the oven and a stew or soup was started in a kettle or Dutch oven cooking pot using the heat from the fireplace. Stews and soups were made once a week and re-boiled daily to make them last without refrigeration. Finally, the week's supply of butter was churned and any other food-related tasks for the week were completed.

Franklin was a believer in order, organization, and schedule. *"Let all your Things have their Places. Let each Part of your Business have its Time,"* he advised. Planning a designated baking day is a smart way to save time during your busy week. Choose one day a week to do your shopping and baking. Make a thorough list before you go to the store to ensure that you've got everything you need. Once the shopping is done, prepare the food that you'll be eating throughout the week.

There are some foods you'll want to prepare on a daily basis, such as oatmeal, rice, and puddings. But with your bread, butter, meal-replacement bars, and soup or stew out of the way, you'll have the majority of your food ready and you won't have to think about it for the rest of the week.

STICK TO THE GUIDELINES AND YOU'LL BE FINE

By sticking to the guidelines of the Ben Franklin Diet, you're stepping onto the road leading to a long and healthy life. You don't have to be seriously strict about every bite of food you put into your mouth, but you will need to be consistent with the quality and quantity of what you eat.

Franklin wrote, *"Never spare the parson's wine, nor the baker's pudding,"* meaning that it's okay to indulge every once in a while, just don't make a habit out of it.

Good luck and happy eating!

Poor Richard, 1733.

AN

Almanack

For the Year of Christ

1733,

PART THREE

Recipes

Being the First after LEAP YEAR:

	Years
And makes since the Creation	7241
By the Account of the Eastern Greeks	6932
By the Latin Church, when O ent. Y	5742
By the Computation of W.W.	5682
By the Roman Chronology	5494
By the Jewish Rabbies	

Wherein is contained

The Lunations, Eclipses, Judgment of the Weather, Spring Tides, Planets Motions & mutual Aspects, Sun and Moon's Rising and Setting, Length of Days, Time of High Water, Fairs, Courts, and observable Days.

Fitted to the Latitude of Forty Degrees, and a Meridian of Five Hours West from *London*, but may without sensible Error, serve all the adjacent Places, even from *Newfoundland* to *South-Carolina.*

By RICHARD SAUNDERS, Philom.

PHILADELPHIA:

Printed and sold by B. FRANKLIN, at the New Printing-Office near the Market.

Introduction to Colonial Cooking

*T*he recipes in this book are for authentic colonial fare. Because recipes of the time were recorded as vague guidelines rather than precise instructions, the original recipes have been reworked and tested to ensure an accurate and delicious outcome for every dish. Meals were traditionally prepared in large pots hanging within the fireplace of the home. The recipes in this book utilize modern cooking appliances to make preparation easy and foolproof.

The goal of the Ben Franklin Diet is to nourish the body and get on with life. Although the simple food is quite pleasant, this book is not about eating for pleasure, it's about *eating to live*. You'll find this sensible diet gives you energy and vigor. Ailments will disappear, and if you're overweight you will slim down and feel a surge of energy you haven't felt in years.

Times have changed, and so have diets. Life is faster paced, people do not take time to focus on their health, the diet suffers, and as a result they are tired, overweight, and have obesity-related diseases, such as diabetes, heart disease, and high blood pressure. It's time to realize that much of the food ingested today is making people sick and, unfortunately for some Americans, their diets contributed to the diseases that led to their deaths.

These recipes are all about getting back to the basics: Whole grains, fruits, and vegetables, with animal products used as accents to the meal, not the main focus. The whole grains provide your body with the necessary carbohydrates and energy you need to live, breathe, think, and exercise. Carbohydrates are *not* the reason Americans are overweight. In fact, eliminating or restricting carbohydrates often leads to intense sugar cravings and bingeing on such sweets as cookies or chocolate. And this, of course, contributes to weight gain so the vicious yo-yo dieting circle starts all over again.

With these recipes and this diet approach, you can satisfy your hunger and sugar cravings with the best, most optimal fuel for your body—whole-grain carbohydrates. Carbohydrates do not make you fat. Excessive calories make you fat. Whether the calories come from soda, juice, chicken, or cookies, consuming more calories than you burn through daily activities, basal metabolism, and exercise, causes weight gain.

—Lisa DeFazio, M.S., R.D.

11

Whole Grains

OATMEAL

If there's one thing to do right off the bat, that's to replace whatever you're eating for breakfast with a bowl of oatmeal, Ben Franklin's favorite breakfast. According to new scientific research studies, this turns out to have been a wise choice for him indeed. It's widely stated that oatmeal *sticks to the ribs*, and current clinical studies show this old saying isn't far from the truth. Besides nourishing the body, oatmeal can help you lose weight. A research study conducted by a cardiologist at Rippe Lifestyle Institute in Orlando, Florida, found that eating oatmeal and losing weight go hand in hand. Forty overweight people were put on a light exercise program and walked for fifteen to thirty minutes per day. Half of the test group was also put on a slightly reduced-calorie diet, which included a bowl of oatmeal for breakfast. The group that ate the oatmeal lost an average of five pounds in the first four weeks, while the other half of the group didn't lose any weight. Although both groups were walking every day, the oatmeal group lost body fat. Over twelve weeks, those who continued walking and eating oatmeal for breakfast lost an average of ten pounds.

Another study conducted by the New York Obesity Center found that eating oatmeal satiates the appetite. Researchers hypothesized that the fiber in the oatmeal slows down the rate at which the stomach empties, in effect making you feel full for long periods of time. Test subjects were given either oatmeal, sugared corn flakes, or water for breakfast. The oatmeal eaters in the study ate 30 percent less at lunch than those in the cereal and water-test groups.

Eating whole oats is one of the most effective ways to reduce cholesterol and the risk of heart attack and heart disease because whole oats have a high proportion of soluble fiber that helps reduce artery-clogging cholesterol. Oatmeal acts a a sponge that soaks up extra cholesterol and helps the body eliminate it, so a bowl of oatmeal in the morning can reduce your cholesterol by up to 20 percent, which translates to a 40-percent reduction in heart-attack risk. Oatmeal is the best breakfast you can eat and is highly recommended as part of the Ben Franklin Diet.

The Two Types of Oatmeal

Both rolled oats and steel-cut oats are whole-grain products. The difference is in how they're processed. Rolled oats are rolled flat and require only a short amount of cooking time because the oats absorb water quickly. During processing, rolled oats are steamed to speed up absorption when water is added to them. Most rolled oats can be added to boiling water and be ready to eat in about five minutes.

Steel-cut oats are made by cutting the whole oat grain into small pieces. These oats usually require longer cooking time (about thirty minutes), but the result is a chunky, chewy oatmeal. Steel-cut oats are also called Scottish or Irish oats because this is the type of oatmeal eaten in the United Kingdom. Quick cooking steel-cut oats that are ready in about five to seven minutes are available in some grocery and health food stores—a great choice if you're in a hurry in the morning.

Which Oat Is Healthier?

Because steel-cut oats have gone through less processing, the oat is closer to its natural state than rolled oats. But both types are equally beneficial and almost identical in nutritional value, so it's a matter of preference. When you buy oats, make sure that, whichever type you choose, they are 100-percent whole and organic. Cooking steel-cut oats takes longer than rolled oats, but the fiber content is slightly higher and this will accelerate weight loss.

For best results in cooking oatmeal, follow the instructions on the package.

Uses for Leftover Oatmeal

If you have leftover oatmeal, don't throw it out. It can be used in other recipes. For example, it can be made especially tasty if it is added to fruit and served with sugar and a little cream. Fruits, such as apples, apricots, berries, fresh bananas, or ripe peaches, may be used for this purpose.

Another way of using leftover oatmeal is to pour it into a pan or a dish and press it down until it is about one inch thick. Then cut it into small pieces, brown the pieces in butter, and serve them with a dash of real maple syrup. Leftover oatmeal can also be served with a baked apple; place a spoonful in a dish with a baked apple, sprinkle a little cinnamon or nutmeg over it, and serve it with a dash of cream.

CORN

The first settlers relied on Indian corn, which remained a staple in the early American diet throughout the seventeenth century. Before there was paper and coin money in the colonies, corn was so valuable that it was used as money. Settlers traded corn with the Indians for wild game, pelts, and other goods. As time went on, the colonists developed new ways of cultivating and preparing corn and cornmeal, eventually combining the grain with other ingredients to make porridge, bread, and a number of different foods, many of which are still popular today.

In 1766, a British writer for the *Gazetteer* and *New Daily Advertiser* had snidely written that American colonists couldn't digest their breakfasts of Indian corn without imported British tea. In defense of corn, Benjamin Franklin wrote to the paper, *"Pray, let me, an American, inform the gentleman, who seems quite ignorant of the matter, that Indian corn, take it for all in all, is one of the most agreeable and wholesome grains in the world; that its green ears roasted are a delicacy beyond expression; that samp, hominy, succatash, nokehock, made of it, are so many pleasing varieties; and that a johnny or hoecake, hot from the fire, is better than a Yorkshire muffin."*

Hasty Pudding

*Hasty pudding, also known as cornmeal mush, is mentioned
numerous times throughout Franklin's writings, and was one
of his favorite meals. Besides being filling and hearty, hasty
pudding costs just pennies to make—a meal for the truly frugal.
For variety, try it for breakfast instead of oatmeal, and add
a little milk and sugar for a hasty, and tasty, meal.*

INGREDIENTS

$1/2$ cup cornmeal

3 cups water

Salt to taste

INSTRUCTIONS

Boil water and add cornmeal. Lower the heat and simmer for
about fifteen minutes, stirring frequently to prevent scorching.
Add salt to taste and serve.

Makes two 1-cup servings

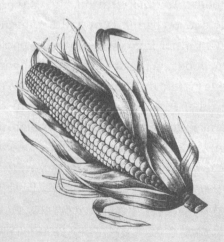

Colonial Corn Custard

This delicious colonial favorite is made with corn, eggs, and milk. Somewhat resembling a quiche, this custard makes a fine and filling meal and is especially nice for breakfast.

INGREDIENTS

4 eggs

2 cups whole milk

$1/4$ cup whole-wheat flour

$2^1/_2$ cups corn kernels
(canned, fresh, or frozen)

2 tablespoons melted butter

1 tablespoon raw sugar

1 teaspoon salt

$1/_2$ teaspoon pepper

INSTRUCTIONS

Preheat the oven to 350 degrees. Beat the eggs with the milk and flour and set aside. Combine all other ingredients in a bowl and stir until mixed. Add the egg/milk/flour mixture and stir until blended. Transfer mixture to a greased baking dish. Set the baking dish on a cookie sheet and bake for 60–65 minutes or until a knife inserted in the center comes out clean.

Makes five 1-cup servings

Real Popcorn

In not much more time than it takes to throw a bag of popcorn into the microwave, you can make your own 100-percent natural popcorn without preservatives and chemicals. Since the introduction of the microwave oven in the 1970s, many people have never tasted real stovetop popcorn. Homemade popcorn seasoned with real butter and sea salt is a delight the entire family will enjoy.

INGREDIENTS

1/4 cup cooking oil

1/2 cup popcorn kernels

Butter (to taste)

Sea salt (to taste)

VARIATIONS

Try experimenting with flavors and seasonings. Adding black pepper, garlic, cinnamon, or other spices can create unique popcorn flavors.

INSTRUCTIONS

Put the oil in the bottom of a large 4-quart pot and add the popcorn. Stir the popcorn to coat the grains with oil. Turn the stove to medium-high heat and put a lid on the pot. When you hear the first kernels popping, shake the pan gently over the stove to avoid burning the kernels. As soon as the popping starts to die down, remove pot from the heat. While the popcorn is still hot, add melted butter and salt to taste.

Makes 8 cups

Brown Rice

*"Rice is known to be one of the best Sorts of Food we have,"
Franklin wrote. "Some whole Provinces, and even
Kingdoms are nourished by it."*

*Brown rice is an excellent staple in any diet. Nearly half
the world's population eats rice every day, especially in India,
China, Japan, and Southeast Asia. Brown rice is a whole grain
with a firm, chewy texture. This whole grain gets its light
brown coloring from the high-fiber bran coating, and this fiber
makes for a very filling meal. USDA researchers discovered that
brown rice is the only grain containing vitamin E, which means
that eating brown rice is beneficial to your skin and to all your
body's cells. Every cup of brown rice also has 4 grams of protein,
and steaming it is the best way to ensure you're getting the
maximum nutrients from the grain.*

INGREDIENTS

I cup of brown rice

2 cups of water

Salt, to taste

INSTRUCTIONS

Rinse and drain the rice. Put the rice and salt in a large pot with
the water and bring to a boil. Once water reaches the boiling
point, remove the pot from heat and cover with a lid. Allow the
rice to steam for 30 minutes. When the rice is done, all the water
in the pot will be gone and the grains will be firm and tender.
Fluff and serve.

Makes $1^1/_2$ cups

RICE

Benjamin Franklin recommended preparing rice several ways: plain, served with butter, served with a small amount of meat, or served with milk poured over it.

Benjamin's Barley Casserole

This delicious casserole can be eaten alone or as a side dish with stew or whole-grain bread. Made with ingredients that were readily available in Colonial America, this recipe offers a little taste of history that's perfectly balanced for use on the Ben Franklin Diet.

INGREDIENTS

$1/2$ cup dried pearl barley	I large chopped onion
$1/2$ cup dried wild rice	I cup sliced mushrooms
6 tablespoons butter	$2^1/_2$ cups chicken broth

INSTRUCTIONS

Preheat oven to 350 degrees. Sauté the barley, wild rice, and 2 tablespoons butter in a large pan over medium heat for 5 minutes. Add the chopped onion, mushrooms, and remaining butter to the pan with the rice and barley and sauté until the onion and mushrooms are tender. Transfer ingredients to a casserole dish, add one cup of chicken broth and place in the preheated oven for 30 minutes. After 30 minutes, add the remaining chicken broth, stir ingredients, and cook for an additional 60 minutes, or until rice and barley are tender.

Makes six 1-cup portions

TABLE OF QUANTITIES
FOR COOKED GRAINS

Following is a table of some of the most commonly cooked whole grains. Half a cup of dry grain weighs approximately 3 ounces and when cooked yields less than one pint—one pint is equal to 2 cups. The idea is to stick to 1-pint portions.

Example: If you cook $^1/_2$ cup of dry oatmeal for breakfast, your cooked grains will yield $1^3/_4$ cups, just $^1/_4$ cup shy of 1 pint. Make up the extra $^1/_4$ cup with some fresh fruit, whole milk, or an easily digestible meat, such as turkey.

Grain, $^1/_2$ Cup Dry	Water	Cooking Time	Yield
Barley	$1^1/_2$ c.	45 minutes	$1^3/_4$ c.
Brown rice	1 c.	60 minutes	$1^1/_2$ c.
Cornmeal	2 c.	25 minutes	$1^1/_2$ c.
Millet	$1^1/_2$ c.	45 minutes	$1^3/_4$ c.
Oats	2 c.	25 minutes	$1^3/_4$ c.
Wheat berries	$1^1/_2$ c.	120 minutes	$1^1/_3$ c.

12

Whole-grain Breads

"Hunger never saw bad bread."
—BEN FRANKLIN

*B*aking your own bread is fun and easy and there's lots of room to get creative with your loaves. Once you get the hang of the basic baking techniques, you can experiment by adding nuts, extra whole grains, onions, garlic, or spices to your bread. While it may sound like a lot of trouble to go to, after you've given it a try and tasted the results, you may never go back to eating store-bought bread again. If taste alone isn't enough to entice you to try baking your own bread, then maybe this will convince you: I lost more weight when I ate homemade bread than when I ate store-bought bread.

BAKING BREAD VERSUS BUYING IT

While many wholesome, 100-percent whole-grain breads can be purchased at the health food or grocery store, it is preferable to grind your own grains and bake bread at home. Besides being economical, you'll discover there's nothing like a loaf of homemade bread fresh from the oven. When you learn the ins and outs of it, baking your own bread becomes a simple, pleasurable task. Additionally, by grinding your own whole grains into flour, you'll get the maximum nutrition from your food. When you buy flour that's already ground, some of the flavor and nutrients have been lost in the process. Grinding fresh flour to bake your breads immediately is ideal, but if you can't find the time to grind and bake, high-quality bread from a natural food store or farmer's market will have to do.

ALL BREADS ARE NOT EQUAL

Homemade, whole-grain breads are dense and tend to weigh more than store-bought whole-grain varieties. When you're eating bread at meals, weigh your slices on a small scale to get an idea of how much grain you're getting. Typically, one slice of homemade bread will outweigh 2 slices of store-bought whole-grain bread. A 4 or 5-ounce portion of bread is equivalent to about 1 cup or half a pint. Weigh your portions until you're familiar enough with them to accurately estimate their weight.

A BRIEF HISTORY OF BREAD

The Essentials of Cookery explains the important relationship between man and bread throughout history and why making bread is vital to good health.

Bread is sometimes defined as any form of baked flour, but as the word is commonly understood it means only those forms of baked flour that contain some leavening substance that produces fermentation. The making of bread has come down through the ages from the simplest methods practiced by the most primitive peoples to the more elaborate processes of the present day. In truth, studying the history of breadmaking would amount to researching accounts of all the progress that has been made by the human race. Still, in order to fully understand the production of bread from suitable ingredients, it will be well to note the advancement that has been made.

In the earliest times, primitive people made what was considered bread in much the same way as today. The grain was ground between stones, usually by hand, then mixed with water to form a dough; and this dough was formed into flat, compact cakes and baked in hot ashes, resulting in a food that was very difficult to digest. Later, someone discovered that by allowing the dough to stand until fermentation took place and then mixing it with new dough, the whole mass would rise, and also that by subjecting this mass to the action of heat, that is, baking it, the mass would be held in place and become a loaf of raised bread that was lighter and, of course, more digestible. It was this discovery that led up to the modern breadmaking processes, in which substances known as leavening agents, or ferments, are used to make bread light, or porous. Chief among these substances is yeast, a microscopic plant that produces fermentation under favorable conditions.

This ferment is so important that, in the United States, whenever the term *bread* is used alone it means yeast, or leavened, bread, whereas, when other leavening agents are used, the bread is referred to as hot bread, or quick bread.

References in the history of the ancient Hebrews show that bread made light by means of fermentation was known thousands of years ago, but it was not until after the accidental discovery of yeast's action that the making of wholesome and digestible bread became possible. With this important advance in the making of bread came a demand for better grains and more improved methods of making flour. Indeed, so much attention has been given to these matters that, at present, the three important processes relating to breadmaking: the raising of wheat, the milling of flour, and the manufacture of yeast; are all carefully and scientifically performed. These industries, together with the commercial manufacture of bread, occupy an important place in the business of practically all civilized nations.

Among people whose cultures are not highly advanced, bread is the chief food and often almost the entire diet, even at the present time; but as mankind progresses, it seems to require a greater variety of food, and devises means of getting that. Since bread is only one of the many foods people find at their disposal, it does not assume as much importance in present-day meals as it formerly did.

Although it does not have the extensive use it had in the past, bread of some description, whether in the form of loaves, biscuits, or rolls, forms a part of each meal in every household. This fact shows that, with the exception of milk, it is more frequently eaten than any other food. If it is properly made, this constantly used food very largely contributes to the family's health.

The Two Types of Bread

When it comes to baking your own breads, there are two types: yeast bread and quick bread. Breads made with yeast, a live organism, must be combined with the other ingredients of the dough and set aside to rise or increase in volume. Then the bread must be kneaded before baking. The process of rising takes 1–1$\frac{1}{2}$ hours before the bread is baked. Quick breads are simply mixed and baked, much like a cake batter, without kneading or waiting for the dough to rise. Recipes for both yeast breads and quick breads are listed in this book and both types were popular in Colonial America.

Tip: Before baking yeast breads, it is important to test your yeast to ensure that it is active. This is called *proofing.* When you combine the yeast with warm water or liquid and sugar in a bowl, the yeast will look slightly foamy and have a distinct yeast smell if it is active and working properly.

Note: The portion size for most of the bread recipes in this book will say eight 5 ounce (one-cup) portions. This means that if you were to cut a loaf of your homemade bread into eight thick slices, each would be the correct size for the Ben Franklin Diet. The weight of the slices will depend on the recipe, but the size is equivalent to about one cup per serving or half a pint.

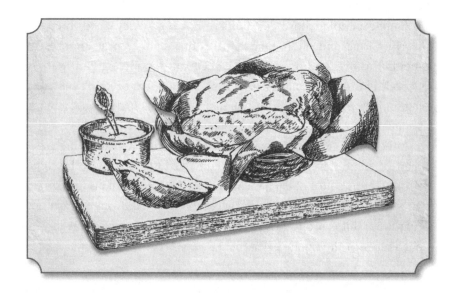

YEAST BREADS

Colonial Sally Lunn Bread

It is believed that this bread was originally called soleil lune,
*French for sun and moon. This recipe makes a basic loaf of delicious,
everyday bread. Sally Lunn bread is a good recipe to try if this
is your first time baking bread. Follow the instructions
precisely and you can't go wrong.*

INGREDIENTS

1 tablespoon active dry yeast	$1/2$ cup melted butter
$1/3$ cup raw sugar	3 eggs
$1/2$ cup warm water	1 teaspoon salt
$1/2$ cup warm milk	4 cups whole-wheat flour

INSTRUCTIONS

Combine yeast, sugar, and warm water in a mixing bowl and stir until
sugar is dissolved. Add milk, butter, eggs, and salt, and stir until mixed.
Add in the flour a little at a time and stir well. Place dough in a greased
bowl and cover with a damp cloth. Let the dough sit in a warm place
and rise for about an hour.

Spread some flour on a flat surface and place the risen dough on it.
Knead the dough back down to its original bulk. Shape into a loaf and
transfer dough into a greased loaf pan and cover it with a damp cloth.
Let the dough sit for another thirty minutes. Bake the bread at 350
degrees for 45 minutes or until a knife inserted in the center of the
loaf comes out clean. Slice and eat.

Makes eight 5-ounce (one-cup) servings

Classic Colonial Bread

*This bread has a crispy crust and a melt-in-your-mouth center.
Made with whole-wheat flour and sea salt, this type of
bread was a staple in the colonial American diet.*

INGREDIENTS

$1^1/_2$ cups warm water

1 tablespoon dry active yeast

2 teaspoons raw sugar

$3^1/_2$ cups whole-wheat flour

2 teaspoons sea salt

1 egg white (to be brushed on top of loaf before baking)

1 tablespoon cornmeal, for baking

INSTRUCTIONS

Combine warm water, yeast, and sugar in a bowl and stir until sugar is
dissolved. Let it sit for about five minutes. In a separate bowl, combine
flour and salt. Add the flour to the yeast water and mix with your hands
until blended. Transfer the dough to a floured surface and knead for
about ten minutes. Transfer the dough into a greased bowl, cover with
a dish towel and let it rise in a warm place for one hour or until the
dough has doubled in bulk. When the dough has risen, knead it again
until it is back to its original bulk. Roll the dough into a long, oval-
shaped loaf and make several sideways slashes across the top of the loaf
with a knife. Brush the loaf with egg white. Transfer the loaf to an
ungreased cookie sheet that has been sprinkled with cornmeal and place
it in a cold oven. Turn the oven on to 400 degrees and let the bread bake
for 30–35 minutes or until the crust is golden brown.

Do not preheat the oven. The gradual increase in temperature bakes
this bread perfectly.

Makes eight 5-ounce (1-cup) servings

Colonial Chesterfield Wheat Bread

This recipe, courtesy of the Hawk's Head Tavern in Oak Glen, California, makes a delicious and authentic loaf of sweet, colonial-era wheat bread. A generous amount of honey gives this dense bread a sweet flavor that patrons of the tavern love.

INGREDIENTS

1 $2/_3$ cup lukewarm water

$1/_2$ cup honey

$1/_4$ cup corn oil

1 tablespoon dry active yeast

3 $1/_3$ cups whole-wheat flour

2 teaspoons salt

INSTRUCTIONS

Preheat oven to 375 degrees. Combine warm water with oil and honey and mix in yeast. Let the mixture sit for about five minutes. Start adding flour one cup at a time, stirring and mixing well. Add in the salt after all of the flour has been added. Cover the bowl with a dishtowel and let it rise in a warm place for one hour or until the dough has doubled in size. When the dough has risen, transfer it to a floured surface and knead until it is back to its original bulk. Roll the dough into a round, somewhat flat loaf and place on a floured cookie sheet. Bake in an oven for 40–50 minutes or until the crust is golden brown and a knife inserted in the center comes out clean.

Makes eight 5-ounce (1-cup) servings

Rye Bread

Rye flour was commonly used in colonial baking. This recipe makes a delicious loaf of old-fashioned rye bread. The flavor is mild, making this hearty bread a perfect accompaniment to a cup of soup.

*For spicy rye bread, add ¼ cup of caraway seeds to the dough before baking.

INGREDIENTS

I cup and 2 tablespoons water

I tablespoon dry active yeast

2 tablespoons raw sugar

2 cups whole-wheat flour

I cup rye flour

2 teaspoons sea salt

2 tablespoons melted butter

INSTRUCTIONS

Preheat oven to 400 degrees. Warm the water and add yeast and sugar, stirring until dissolved. In a separate bowl, combine the flours and salt and stir until blended. Pour the water and yeast mixture into the flour and stir until mixed. Add melted butter and work into the dough. Flour a hard surface and knead dough for a few minutes until springy. Transfer dough to a greased bowl. Cover with a kitchen towel and set in a warm place for about an hour or until dough has doubled in bulk. Flour a hard surface again and knead dough until it's back to original bulk before rising. Shape into a loaf and place it in a greased, floured loaf pan. Cover pan with a kitchen towel and let it rise again for another 30 minutes. Put the loaf pan in the preheated over and bake for 30 minutes. Slice and serve.

Makes eight 5-ounce (1-cup) servings

QUICK BREADS

Colonial Buttermilk Bread

This classic Colonial American recipe makes one loaf of delicious sweet bread. No yeast or kneading is called for because the buttermilk and soda react to make it rise. This tasty bread is very versatile and you may experiment by replacing up to one cup of the whole-wheat flour with the flour of your choice, such as oat, rice, or bran.

INGREDIENTS

3 cups whole-wheat flour

$1/2$ cup brown sugar

2 teaspoons baking soda

1 teaspoon sea salt

2 cups buttermilk

INSTRUCTIONS

Preheat oven to 350 degrees. Combine flour, sugar, baking soda, and salt and stir until blended. Pour in the buttermilk and stir until well mixed. Spoon dough into a greased and floured pan and bake for 1 hour or until a knife inserted in the center comes out clean. Serve warm.

Makes eight 4-ounce (1-cup) servings

Benjamin Franklin's Maize and Whole Wheat Cornbread

Benjamin Franklin was a fan of cornbread. In an unpublished letter, originally written in French, he wrote instructions to make cornbread using water, ground Indian maize (cornmeal), and wheat flour.

> *"Corn flour requires more time to cook than the wheat flour. Therefore, if they are mixed together cold at the initial stage and allowed to ferment and cook, the wheat part will be cooked when the corn part will still be raw.*
>
> *"To overcome this drawback, we boil a pot of water. While water is boiling, throw a little salt in with one hand, [and] some corn flour while stirring with the other. This process should be repeated with a little flour each time until the mass becomes so thick that it is difficult to stir with a stick. Then, after some time, while it is still left on the fire, until the last handful of corn has been boiled, remove it, and pour the mass into the bread bin, where it must be well mixed and kneaded with a quantity of wheat flour sufficient enough to form a dough good enough for bread. Then any leaven or beer leaven is needed to make the dough rise. After the necessary time, mold, shape and put bread in the oven."*

Cornbread was one of the first breads eaten in Colonial America. It was sometimes made by travelers and carried on long journeys. Cornbread was ideal for long trips because it didn't spoil easily and provided good nutrition. People began to call cornbread "journey cake" from which came the name

"Johnny Cake." Traditionally made with cornmeal, flour, eggs, butter, and sugar, cornbread, or Johnny cake, is still a popular bread today.

Because Benjamin Franklin's instructions for making cornbread were vague, as were most colonial recipes, the following recipe using cornmeal and whole-wheat flour was created so you can make a loaf of this delicious bread.

INGREDIENTS

$3/4$ cup yellow cornmeal

$1^1/_4$ cups whole-wheat flour

2 tablespoons raw sugar

$1/_2$ teaspoon salt

I tablespoon baking powder

I cup whole milk

I egg

2 tablespoons melted butter

INSTRUCTIONS

Preheat oven to 350 degrees. Combine the cornmeal, flour, sugar, salt, and baking powder and stir until mixed. Add the milk, egg, and butter, and stir until well blended. Pour into a greased and floured 9 x 9 square pan and bake for about 30 minutes or until a knife in the center comes out clean. Cut into 8 pieces and serve warm.

Makes eight 4-ounce (1-cup) servings

Hoecakes

A hoecake is a simple bread made with cornmeal. Traditionally, this bread was made while traveling and baked over an open fire on the back of a hoe or metal shovel. Benjamin Franklin loved hoecakes, and in a letter printed in the Gazetteer *newspaper he wrote, in defense of Indian corn,* "a johnny or a hoecake, hot from the fire, is better than a Yorkshire muffin."

INGREDIENTS

I cup cornmeal	I teaspoon raw sugar
$1/2$ cup whole milk	I cup water
I tablespoon softened butter	Pinch of salt

INSTRUCTIONS

Combine all ingredients in a pot and stir until blended. Cook over medium heat, stirring constantly until mixture becomes a thick dough, about 3 minutes. Remove from heat and let the dough cool. When cool enough to handle, divide dough into 8 egg-sized balls. Flatten the balls in the palm of your hand so they are about 4 inches round. Add a little butter to a large frying pan and cook four hoecakes at a time over medium-high heat. Cook them on one side until lightly browned (about 4 minutes), then flip them over and brown the other side (about 4 minutes). Serve with a pat of butter and a drizzle of honey or maple syrup on top. Hoecakes make a delicious breakfast. Makes eight 4" cakes

Makes eight 2.5-ounce ($1/2$-cup) servings

VARIATIONS

Add a $1/4$ cup of diced onions to the batter for a delicious onion flavor, or add $1/4$ cup of fresh corn kernels to the batter for a chunkier texture.

Irish Soda Bread

Irish Soda Bread is simple to make and requires just a few basic ingredients. This old-fashioned recipe makes one small loaf of bread that is crispy on the outside and moist on the inside.

INGREDIENTS

2 cups whole-wheat flour

$^3/_4$ cup all-purpose flour

1 tablespoon raw sugar

1 teaspoon baking soda

$^1/_2$ teaspoon salt

1 cup buttermilk

INSTRUCTIONS

Preheat oven to 425 degrees. Combine flour, sugar, baking soda, and salt in a large bowl and stir until blended. Add the buttermilk to form a sticky dough. Continue mixing and kneading the dough with your hands until you've formed a ball. Place dough on a floured cookie sheet. Cut a large *X* across the top of the loaf with a knife. Bake for 35–40 minutes or until the crust is golden brown and a knife inserted in the center comes out clean. To keep your soda bread moist, cover it with a kitchen towel or tea towel until ready to serve. Slice bread into 4 triangular slices as you would a pie.

Makes four 5-ounce (1-cup) servings

VARIATION

Sweet Raisin Soda Bread. To make a sweeter, raisin variety of Irish Soda Bread, add an additional 2 tablespoons of raw sugar and $^1/_2$ cup raisins to the recipe above.

Colonial Gingerbread

Spicy gingerbread was a popular remedy for seasickness in colonial times. Benjamin Franklin wrote of purchasing loaves from the baker before his long ocean journey from Philadelphia to London. A slice of moist, Colonial Gingerbread makes a sweet and spicy meal. Try a slice of this bread warm with a pat of homemade butter.

INGREDIENTS

1/2 cup water (boiling)

1/2 cup brown sugar

1/2 cup molasses

1/2 cup melted butter

I egg

2 tablespoons fresh grated ginger
(vastly superior to the
powdered variety but you can
substitute powdered if necessary)

I tablespoon ground cinnamon

1/4 teaspoon ground cloves

2 cups whole-wheat flour

I teaspoon baking soda

I tablespoon apple cider vinegar

Note: *See* Spices in Chapter 16 for additional
information on ginger.

INSTRUCTIONS

Preheat oven to 325 degrees. Combine sugar, molasses, melted butter, egg, ginger, cinnamon, and cloves in a large bowl and stir until smooth. In a separate bowl, combine flour and baking soda. Pour the boiling water into the flour and stir until mixed. Add the flour mixture to the sugar and molasses mixture and beat until smooth. Add the vinegar and mix a little more. Pour the batter into a greased 9 x 9 square pan and bake for 45–50 minutes or until a knife inserted into the center of the loaf comes out clean.

Let the loaf cool, cut into 8 equal pieces and serve. Wrap unused pieces individually and store in the refrigerator for up to 1 week, or in the freezer for up to 2 months.

Makes eight 4-ounce (1-cup) servings

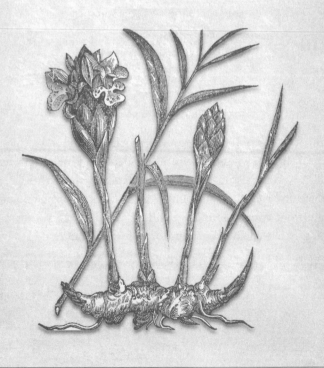

Oatcakes

Oatcakes, known as dietary biscuits in Colonial America, are a simple bread with a slightly chewy texture. Oatcakes were a staple in traditional Scottish and English diets and are still popular today in the United Kingdom. Shaped into small rounds, these delightful little cakes resemble cookies. Oatcakes can be eaten with thin slices of cheese, topped with a bit of whole-fruit preserves, or drizzled with honey or maple syrup.

Note: Perfect as a snack on the Ben Franklin Diet.

INGREDIENTS

1 cup rolled oats

1 cup whole-wheat flour

1 teaspoon baking soda

Pinch of salt

2 tablespoons melted butter

1 cup boiling water

INSTRUCTIONS

Preheat oven to 400 degrees. Combine oats, flour, baking soda, and salt in a bowl and stir until blended. Add melted butter and boiling water, stirring until mixed. Transfer dough to a floured surface and roll it out to about $1/4$ inch thick. Using a cookie cutter, cut out twenty-four 2" rounds. Place all twenty-four rounds on a greased cookie sheet and bake for 10 minutes.

Makes 24 oatcakes; six oatcakes per 4-ounce (1-cup) portion

Boston Brown Bread

It is believed that Boston Brown Bread was the original bread recipe from the American colonies. First made in Boston, thus the name, it quickly gained popularity among people everywhere. Traditionally, this steamed bread was served with baked beans. A generous amount of molasses and raisins gives this loaf a sweet flavor.

INGREDIENTS

$1/2$ cup whole-wheat flour

$1/2$ cup cornmeal

$1/2$ cup rye flour

$1/2$ cup molasses

$1/2$ cup buttermilk

$1/2$ cup raisins

1 teaspoon baking soda

$1/2$ teaspoon salt

INSTRUCTIONS

Combine all ingredients in a bowl and stir until blended. Take a clean 1-pound coffee or vegetable can and grease the inside with butter. Pour the batter into the can and cover the top tightly with aluminum foil. Place the can on top of a rack or trivet inside a large soup pot and fill the pot with enough water to come up to the middle of the outside of the can. Bring the water to a boil. Then lower heat to a simmer, cover the pot, and allow the bread to steam for 2 hours, adding water to the pot, if necessary. Carefully lift the hot can out of the pot and take off the foil. Slide the bread out of the can (removing its bottom with a can opener can facilitate this). Slice and serve.

Makes four 4-ounce (1-cup) servings

Blackberry Walnut Bread

Wild berries such as blackberries grew abundantly in Northern America and were gathered by settlers. The colonists often added fresh fruit and nuts to their bread. This recipe is wonderful served with a pat of butter or a small amount of cream cheese on top. Blackberries are high in vitamin C and antioxidants, making this a nice breakfast bread to start the day with.

INGREDIENTS

2 cups whole-wheat flour

3/4 cup brown sugar

1 teaspoon baking soda

1 1/2 teaspoons baking powder

1 cup unfiltered, unsweetened apple juice

1/3 cup melted butter

1 egg

1 1/2 cups fresh blackberries

1/2 cup chopped walnuts

INSTRUCTIONS

Preheat oven to 350 degrees. Combine flour, sugar, baking soda, and baking powder in a bowl and stir until mixed. In a separate bowl, combine apple juice, melted butter, and egg, and stir until blended. Add juice mixture to flour mixture and stir until smooth. Add blackberries and walnuts and stir. Spoon dough into a greased and floured loaf pan and bake for 55–65 minutes or until knife inserted in the center comes out clean. Let loaf cool, slice, and serve.

Makes eight 5-ounce (1-cup) servings

VARIATION

You may replace the blackberries with fresh raspberries, gooseberries, or blueberries.

Note: If you use frozen blackberries, thaw and drain the juice before adding them to the batter.

Buttermilk Carrot Loaf

Carrots were a popular root vegetable in Colonial America. After the harvest, colonists stored carrots in root cellars and enjoyed this vitamin-packed vegetable all year round. This dark, aromatic carrot cake is packed with freshly grated carrots, whole-grain wheat and wholesome buttermilk. Have a slice with a meal or enjoy a piece or two for breakfast. It's a sweet treat that's good for you.

INGREDIENTS

1 cup whole-wheat flour

1 cup brown sugar

1 teaspoon baking soda

2 teaspoons ground cinnamon

2 eggs

1/4 cup buttermilk

1/4 cup melted butter

1 tablespoon molasses

1 teaspoon vanilla extract

4 cups carrots, grated (about 4 large carrots)

INSTRUCTIONS

Preheat oven to 350 degrees. Combine flour, sugar, soda, and cinnamon in a large bowl and stir until mixed. In a separate bowl combine eggs, buttermilk, melted butter, molasses, and vanilla extract, and stir until blended. Add buttermilk mixture to flour mixture and stir until smooth. Add shredded carrots and stir. Spoon dough into a greased and floured loaf pan and bake for 55 minutes or until knife inserted in the center comes out clean. Let loaf cool, slice, and serve. Store any unused carrot loaf in a sealed container.

Makes eight 5-ounce (1-cup) servings

Benjamin Franklin Meal-Replacement Energy Bars

In 1784, Benjamin Franklin wrote a letter to his friend David LeRoy concerning improvements for traveling by ship. In the letter he provided a list of recommended food items that passengers should carry with them, including almonds, chocolate, eggs, sugar, raisins, rum, and oat bread. I have taken the liberty of turning Franklin's list of rations into succulent whole-grain bars that are perfect for a meal replacement or an energy-packed snack bar. Each bar has 240 calories, 40 grams of carbohydrates, and a full 15 grams of protein. The Benjamin Franklin Meal-Replacement Energy Bars were designed to provide all the whole grain and daily nutrition the body needs. You will lose weight if you eat four to six of these per day instead of meals and snacks. These bars are great if you're on the go and need to have a meal on hand without thinking about it. (Two bars make a pint-sized meal replacement.)

INGREDIENTS

I cup whole milk

2 eggs

$1/4$ cup honey

2 tablespoons unsweetened applesauce

I tablespoon dark rum (or substitute I teaspoon vanilla extract)

$3/4$ cup brown sugar

$1^1/2$ cups whole-wheat flour

I teaspoon ground cinnamon

I teaspoon baking soda

$2^1/2$ cups rolled oats

$1/2$ cup semi-sweet chocolate chips

$1/2$ cup dried cranberries

$1/4$ cup almonds or walnuts, chopped

$1/4$ cup raisins

INSTRUCTIONS

Preheat oven to 350 degrees. In a large bowl, combine milk, eggs, honey, applesauce, rum or vanilla, and sugar. Stir until blended. In a separate bowl, combine flour, cinnamon, and baking soda. Stir until mixed. Add the flour mixture to the milk mixture and stir until blended. Add the oats, chocolate chips, cranberries, almonds, and raisins and stir until blended. Spoon mixture into a greased 9 x 13 pan and smooth out evenly in pan. Bake for 28–30 minutes. Let cool completely and cut into 12 bars. Wrap individual bars in plastic wrap or store in a sealed container

Makes twelve 4-ounce servings

Note: For a delightful treat that's good for you, try one of these bars warmed up with a pat of butter on top.

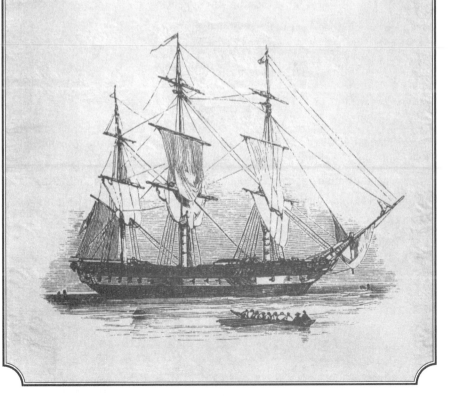

Mrs. Wright's Beer Bread

*This delicious beer bread is easy to make and requires
only five simple ingredients. Low in fat and rich in taste,
this bread utilizes beer as a leavening agent (a popular
ingredient in colonial bread making). To make a
delicately flavored loaf of bread, use light beer.
For a dark, heavier taste, try using a bottle of ale.
You can also use non-alcoholic beer if you wish.*

INGREDIENTS

3 cups whole wheat flour

1/4 cup raw sugar

1 tablespoon baking powder

1 teaspoon sea salt

1 12-ounce bottle of beer or ale

INSTRUCTIONS

Preheat oven to 375 degrees. Combine flour, sugar, baking powder
and salt in a large bowl and stir until blended. Slowly pour in
beer and stir until you have a sticky dough. Spoon dough into
a greased and floured 9" x 5" loaf pan and bake for 35–40 minutes or until a knife inserted in the center comes out clean.
Serve warm.

Makes eight 4-ounce (1-cup) servings

13

Soups and Stews

Soups and stews were popular foods in colonial times. Housewives would prepare soup or stew in a large kettle suspended over the flames of the fireplace where they would simmer overnight. Made with fresh vegetables, herbs, and grains, these liquid meals satisfied even the heartiest of appetites.

Soups and stews make easy meals you can incorporate into your diet. For a simple meal, you can eat 1 pint of soup or stew. If you're looking for variety, eat one cup of soup or stew per meal with 4 ounces of whole-grain bread or 4 ounces of fresh vegetables.

Note: If you have high cholesterol or heart disease or are trying to decrease fat and cholesterol in your diet, substitute whole milk with 2-percent or fat-free milk. Two-percent milk has some fat and this will give you a creamy consistency with less fat.

Colonial
Corn Chowder

*This traditional corn chowder recipe can be enjoyed at lunch
or dinner. It is particularly nice on a chilly day. Enjoy a cup
with a thick slice of homemade bread, or make an entire
meal of this chowder and have a full pint.*

INGREDIENTS

1 pound of fresh or frozen corn kernels,
about 6 ears

3 cups whole milk

2 tablespoons butter

1 teaspoon sea salt

2 teaspoons black pepper

2 tablespoons whole-wheat flour

INSTRUCTIONS

Combine corn, milk, butter, salt, and pepper in a large pot over
medium heat. Stir frequently to avoid scalding. When the butter
is melted, stir in the flour a little at a time until mixture thickens.
Bring to a boil while stirring. Remove from heat and serve.

Makes six 1-cup servings

Pennsylvania Dutch Potato Soup

The Pennsylvania Dutch of the seventeenth century were farming people of German, or Deutsch, *descent who brought their simple cooking ways from the Old World. This soup was traditionally served over cubed brown bread and topped with a piece of crispy, crumbled bacon. Whether you eat the soup by itself or with a slice of bread and bacon, you're sure to enjoy the meal.*

INGREDIENTS

3 cups water (or enough to cover potatoes and onions in pot)

2 large brown potatoes, unpeeled and diced (for a smoother, less rustic-looking soup, peel potatoes before dicing.)

1 yellow onion, peeled and diced

1 cup whole milk

2 teaspoons sea salt

1 teaspoon black pepper

4-ounce slice whole-grain bread, cubed

1 slice crispy bacon (optional)

INSTRUCTIONS

Place diced potatoes and onions in a large pot with water and bring to a boil. Turn the heat down and put a lid on the pot, allowing it to simmer for about 40 minutes or until vegetables are soft. Stir in milk, sour cream, salt, and pepper, and stir with a wire whisk. Remove from heat and pour 1 cup over a cubed slice of brown whole-grain bread. Top with a slice of crispy, crumbled bacon (optional).

Makes eight 1-cup servings

Note: This potato soup makes an excellent base for New England-style clam or seafood chowder. Add 1 cup of cooked clams, fish, or shellfish to this soup for a pot of tasty seafood chowder.

Tom's Split Pea Porridge

In sixteenth-century England and Scotland, a thick porridge made of dried peas was often cooked over the fireplace in the home, especially among the poorer people where meat was scarce. Known as pease porridge, *this thick stew often included ham bones, carrots, onions, garlic, and other available vegetables. Nothing went to waste. This porridge evolved from Pease Pottage, a very thick dish made from dried green peas that was flavored with salted bacon. Thomas Tryon wrote in his 1691 vegetarian cookbook,* "Dry Pease being boiled in plenty of Water, being seasoned with Salt and Butter, makes a substantial Dish of Food, and affords a strong nourishment, and are good for all strong labouring Men." *When the fire was lit each morning, more dried peas, water, and vegetables would be added to the kettle providing a constant supply of hearty soup. Pease porridge was a favorite of Benjamin Franklin's. In fact, when he was visiting England in 1770, he had a shipment of dried green peas sent back to a friend in the colonies. Franklin wrote,* "I send, also, some green dry Pease, highly esteemed here as the best for making pease soup."

INGREDIENTS

1 lb. bag (2¼ cups) dried split green peas

7 cups water

2 cups cooked ham, diced

Ham hock

1 large brown onion, chopped

1 cup celery, chopped

1 cup carrots, chopped

2 cloves garlic, minced

2 bay leaves

Salt and pepper to taste

Parsley for garnish

INSTRUCTIONS

Before cooking, rinse and pick through peas to remove any residue material. (It is not necessary to soak the peas in water before cooking them.) Add peas and water to a large soup pot and bring to a boil. Add chopped ham, ham hock, onion, celery, carrots, garlic, and bay leaves. Cover pot and reduce heat to a simmer, stirring occasionally to prevent the soup from sticking to the bottom of the pot. Let it cook for $1^1/_2$ to 2 hours or until peas are soft. Remove from heat and discard ham hock and bay leaves. Add salt and pepper to taste, garnish with fresh parsley, and serve. Store any leftover soup in the refrigerator or freezer. Leftover soup will thicken overnight.

Makes nine 1-cup servings

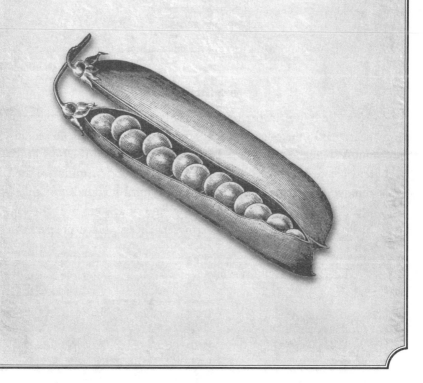

Onion and Ale Soup

This savory soup is made with browned onions and flavored with a splash of ale. Parmesan cheese, one of Benjamin Franklin's favorite foods, tops off this flavorful soup.

INGREDIENTS

2 tablespoons butter

4 yellow or brown onions, thinly sliced

4 cups beef broth

$\frac{1}{4}$ cup ale*

2 teaspoons whole-wheat flour

4 slices whole-grain bread, cubed

Grated Parmesan cheese,
up to 1 oz. per serving

Black pepper and salt, to taste

*If you don't like the flavor of ale, simply delete it from this recipe.

INSTRUCTIONS

Melt the butter in the bottom of a large soup pot over medium heat. Stir in the onions, stirring them frequently to avoid scorching. When the onions are browned and soft, add the beef broth and ale to the pot. Boil the soup for about ten minutes, then remove from heat. Add flour, stirring until blended. Put cubed bread in the bottom of a soup bowl and pour soup over the top. Sprinkle soup with grated Parmesan cheese, black pepper, and salt to taste.

Makes four 1-cup servings

Brunswick Stew

Brunswick Stew is a traditional colonial favorite. This stew was originally made with wild game, squirrel, and rabbit. But as time went on, settlers began to use chicken and pork instead. There are many recipes for this stew, but they all include a tomato base, lima beans, corn, and two kinds of meat, most commonly chicken and pork. The origins of Brunswick Stew vary as well. Some say the first batch of this stew was made in Brunswick County, Virginia, while others believe it was an import from Braunschweig, Germany. Whatever the origin, this stew makes a hearty and delicious meal.

INGREDIENTS

6 cups chicken stock

3 cups of cooked chicken or turkey, cubed

1 28-oz. can diced tomatoes

1 yellow onion, diced

2 cups fresh or frozen lima beans

1 cup fresh or frozen corn kernels

8 pieces of bacon, cooked and crumbled

2 medium potatoes, boiled and mashed

1 teaspoon black pepper

1 bay leaf

INSTRUCTIONS

In a large soup pot, combine chicken stock, cooked chicken, tomatoes, onions, lima beans, and corn, and stir. Turn the heat to simmer. Add the crumbled bacon, mashed potatoes, salt, pepper, and bay leaf. Stir until well mixed. Cover the pot and allow the stew to simmer for 2 hours. If you use a crock pot, cook stew on the low setting for about 3 hours.

Makes sixteen 1-cup portions

Tom's Turkey Soup

This soup recipe is a great way to make good use of your leftover turkey bones and meat. As Benjamin Franklin said, "waste nothing." Tom's Turkey Soup is simple, rustic and delicious.

INGREDIENTS

Bones and leftover meat of 1 turkey

8 cups chicken broth

2 cups water

1 onion, chopped

1 cup celery, chopped

1 cup carrots, chopped

1 cup corn

1 cup dried wild rice

Salt and pepper to taste

INSTRUCTIONS

Place turkey carcass in a large soup pot. Add chicken broth and water and bring to a boil. Add onion, celery, carrots, corn, and dried wild rice, and lower heat. Simmer soup for 2 hours or until rice is tender. Remove turkey bones and carcass from the soup. Add salt and pepper to taste.

Makes fourteen 1-cup servings

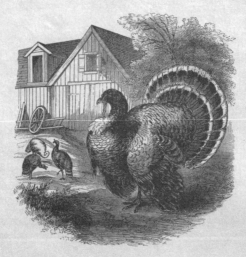

Spicy Pumpkin Soup

Pumpkins were a readily available source of food in the colonies. Pumpkins are large gourds with a sweet flavor. The word pumpkin comes from the French word pompion, which was derived from Greek, meaning "cooked by the sun." These large, sweet gourds are naturally rich in vitamin A and fiber. This spicy pumpkin soup makes a great accompaniment to fresh-baked bread. You may use canned pumpkin, but try this recipe in the fall using a fresh pumpkin for an unforgettably inviting meal. For instructions on how to cook a fresh pumpkin, see the inset on page 128.

INGREDIENTS

$3^1/_2$ cups fresh-cooked pumpkin, pureed
(or a 29-oz. can of pumpkin)

2 cups whole milk

2 cups chicken broth

2 teaspoons sea salt

$^1/_2$ teaspoon nutmeg

$^1/_8$ teaspoon cayenne pepper

1 bunch of green onions

Light sour cream (optional)

INSTRUCTIONS

Combine pumpkin, milk, chicken broth, salt, nutmeg, and cayenne pepper in a large soup pot and stir over medium heat until it comes to a boil. Remove from heat and serve. Top with chopped green onions. Add a tablespoon of sour cream on top the soup, if desired, and add additional cayenne pepper to taste if you like your soup spicier.

Makes six 1-cup servings

Tavern Soup

*Imagine stopping at the tavern for a pint of ale or perhaps a
secret town meeting. You smell the aromatic soup as it bubbles in
a cauldron over the open flames of the fireplace. You are served
a bowl of it with a chunk of bread on the side as you greet your
friends by the flickering candlelight. Inspired by simple colonial
tavern fare, this rustic soup is made with barley and vegetables
in tasty beef broth, combining whole grains and vegetables—
a hearty meal for weary travelers.*

INGREDIENTS

8 cups beef broth

6 large carrots, diced

6 celery stalks, diced

2 large potatoes, unpeeled and diced

2 large yellow onions, diced

1 cup uncooked pearl barley

$1/2$ cup fresh chopped parsley

1 tablespoon sea salt

1 teaspoon ground black pepper

INSTRUCTIONS

Combine all ingredients in a large soup pot and bring to a boil.
Lower heat, cover, and simmer for 45 minutes. Serve with a chunk
of fresh baked bread.

Makes eight 1-cup servings

Note: If you add more vegetables to this soup, increase the
amount of beef broth to ensure that the vegetables are submerged
in liquid.

Benjamin Franklin's Recipe for Dauphiny Soup

Benjamin Franklin published a recipe for Dauphiny Soup in the Farmer's Almanac of 1756. "A Recipe for Dauphiny Soup, which in Turkey is called Touble, and with which a great Number of Persons may be Plentifully fed at a very small Expence," *he wrote.* "This Soup is agreeable to the Taste, very filling and nourishing."

The soup is simple and bland, and most kitchens have all the ingredients on hand to make it in a pinch. This recipe, originally intended to feed a crowd, has been scaled down.

INGREDIENTS

$4^2/_3$ cups water, divided

$1^1/_2$ cups whole-wheat flour

2 teaspoons salt

2 tablespoons butter

INSTRUCTIONS

Combine the flour and 1 teaspoon of salt with $^2/_3$ cups water. Mix it with your hands until you have a ball of dough. On a floured surface, roll the ball flat with a rolling pin until it is about $^1/_4$ inch thick. Slice the dough into $^1/_2$ inch strips and slice the strips into small pieces about $^1/_2$ inch wide. Bring the remaining 4 cups of water, plus 1 teaspoon of salt and the butter to a rolling boil in a large pot. Add the dough pieces. Lower the heat and allow the soup to boil gently for $1^1/_2$ hours. The dough pieces will swell to about twice their original size. Serve the soup while it's hot. Before eating, you can spice it up by adding salt and pepper to taste, and/or grated Parmesan cheese, if you wish.

Makes four 1-cup servings

VEGETABLES AND FRUITS IN COLONIAL AMERICA

Vegetables in Soups

Taverns and inns in Colonial America would make soup for their patrons out of the vegetables they had on hand. Dried grains, such as barley, and root vegetables, including potatoes, carrots, and onions, were usually available. But the soup would change depending on what vegetables were in season. You can add your own fresh, seasonal vegetables, such as broccoli, corn, green beans, or zucchini, to a soup.

VEGETABLE AND FRUIT RECIPES

Outside of soups and stews, there are few recipes for cooking vegetables in this book, and Chapter 15, Sweet Fare, has most of the recipes containing fruit. Overall, the best way to consume vegetables and fruits is in their raw state because cooking leads to nutrient loss and you want to get the maximum amount of nutrition and fiber from every bite you eat.

You can eat one to two cups of fresh vegetables a day, and one cup of fresh fruit a day. Vegetables and fruits can be incorporated into your meals or eaten as snacks. In season, organic produce is preferable.

HOW TO COOK A PUMPKIN

Choose a small, firm *pie* pumpkin about the size of a soccer ball. Cut the pumpkin in half and scrape out all seeds and stringy pulp. Place the two pumpkin halves on a greased cookie sheet and bake at 300 degrees for 1 hour. When you remove the pumpkin halves, the flesh should be soft enough to scrape it from the skin. Place the cooked pumpkin in a bowl and mash it with an electric mixer or a potato masher. Use cooked pumpkin for Spicy Pumpkin Soup, page 125.

14

Meat, Poultry, Fish, and Dairy

MEAT

You may incorporate meat into your daily meals if you like. The human body can easily digest small amounts of meat, such as turkey, chicken, or fish. Benjamin Franklin preferred these white meats over beef, venison, or pork, which made him feel sluggish afterward. If you choose to eat meat, use it as a garnish rather than the main dish, and buy only organic meat. Meat should be eaten in combination with whole grains. Serve chicken, turkey, or fish with whole-grain bread or a bowl of rice for a tasty and satisfying meal. Although it is not necessary to eat meat on the Ben Franklin Diet, it is by no means forbidden. If you do eat meat, keep the portions to three ounces or less per day, which is about the size of a deck of cards.

FISH

Fish is high in healthy, omega-3 essential fatty acids and is considered good for your health as long as you choose wisely and avoid any fish that contain significant levels of mercury. *The American Journal of Clinical Nutrition* found that fish high in omega-3 are known to reduce the risk of diabetes, depression, heart disease, strokes, and some cancers. Fish containing the highest amount of omega-3 are albacore tuna, anchovies, herring, and salmon.

While you can eat canned salmon, tuna, or other fish on the Ben Franklin Diet, it is preferable to eat fresh fish.

How to Cook Fish the Easy Way

The easiest way to cook a fish is in a pan. Begin with a fish fillet. Place a small amount of butter in a medium-hot frying pan and add a little minced garlic if you like. Cook the fish fillet ten minutes for every inch of thickness, turning it once while cooking so that both sides are browned. If your fillet is only a half-inch thick, cook it for five minutes or until the fish starts to separate and get flaky. Serve the fish with brown rice, salad, or soup.

Variations

- Before cooking, you can brush the uncooked fish fillet with a little beaten egg and roll it in bread crumbs and spices, or nuts, such as crushed almonds. This adds a crunchy outer crust.

- After cooking, you can sprinkle some fresh lemon juice over the cooked fish and eat.

POULTRY—CHICKEN AND TURKEY

Chicken or turkey are great sources of protein that are easy to prepare and versatile enough to be used in many different meals. You can cook ahead of time and keep the cooked meat in the refrigerator to use in recipes throughout the week. Cooked chicken or turkey breasts can be sliced up and added to soups and salads, or made into chicken/turkey salad for sandwiches.

Sautéed Chicken Breasts

The easiest way to cook chicken breasts is to sauté them. Add a small amount of butter or olive oil to the sauté pan, turn the heat up to medium, and lay the chicken breasts flat. If you like, you can add some minced garlic, salt, pepper, or other spices to suit your taste. Let the chicken breasts cook on one side for three to four minutes, then flip them over and let the other side cook for about three to four minutes.

Note: Because breast thickness varies, cut into the breasts before removing them from the pan to ensure they have cooked all the way through.

Chicken Pot Pie

This recipe makes 4 delectable individual chicken pot pies in true colonial style. With a whole-grain crust, tender vegetables, and a creamy sauce, these pies are worth the trouble.

INGREDIENTS FOR FILLING

2 cups cooked chicken, cubed

3 tablespoons butter

1 potato, diced

2 carrots, diced

1 onion, minced

2 cups chicken broth

4 tablespoons whole-wheat flour

2 teaspoons sea salt

$1/2$ cup whole milk

INSTRUCTIONS

Melt butter in a large pot over medium heat. Add potatoes, carrots, and onion and stir gently for about ten minutes. Add the chicken broth and allow mixture to come to a boil. Lower heat to a simmer and stir in flour, salt, and milk, stirring until sauce is creamy. Cook, stirring constantly, for 10 minutes, then remove from heat, add the chicken, and set aside while you make the pie crust.

INGREDIENTS FOR CRUST

$1^{1}/_{2}$ cups whole-wheat flour

1 teaspoon sea salt

$1/2$ cup butter

4 tablespoons ice water

INSTRUCTIONS

Preheat oven to 400 degrees. Put flour into a large bowl and stir in salt. Cut butter into small pieces and add it to flour. Using your fingers, crush the butter pieces into the flour mixture. Add ice water and continue mixing the flour with your hands. Form it into a ball. Place the dough ball on a floured surface and roll it out flat to about $1/_8$ inch thick. Spoon the pot pie filling into four oven-safe crocks or miniature pie pans and fill $1/_2$ an inch below the edge. Cut out four pieces of pie crust and lay them over the top of each dish. Pinch and press the pie crust dough around the edges of each dish and cut two 1-inch slits in the center of each pie-crust top. Place pies in the oven and bake for 20 minutes. Remove from oven and serve.

Makes four 2-cup servings

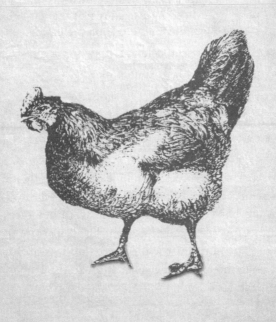

Baked Turkey Hotpot

*This one-dish recipe combines the best of a traditional
Thanksgiving dinner, including cranberries, stuffing, and
tender, delicious turkey. This tasty meal is packed
with whole grains and can be eaten anytime.*

INGREDIENTS

$1^1/_2$ cups chicken broth

2 tablespoons melted butter

1 teaspoon sea salt

$^1/_2$ teaspoon ground thyme

$^1/_2$ teaspoon ground sage

$^1/_2$ teaspoon black pepper

6 cups whole-grain bread, cubed

1 pound uncooked turkey-breast tenders,
approximately 1 turkey breast,
sliced into small pieces
(substitute chicken if you prefer)

1 cup celery, chopped

1 large onion, diced

$^1/_2$ cup dried cranberries

$^1/_2$ cup apple cider

INSTRUCTIONS

Preheat oven to 350 degrees. Combine chicken broth, melted butter, salt, thyme, sage, and pepper in a bowl and stir until blended. In a separate bowl, combine bread cubes, turkey pieces, celery, onion, and cranberries and toss. Pour broth mixture over bread mixture and stir until mixed. Place mixture in a greased baking dish and pour the apple cider over it. Bake for 1 hour. Remove from oven and serve.

Makes eight 1-cup servings

Tom's Roasted Herb Turkey

Roasted turkey was a mainstay of the colonial diet. With plenty of wild turkeys, colonists dined regularly on this large bird. Don't wait until the holidays to enjoy turkey. It makes a great meal anytime of the year.

INGREDIENTS

1 fresh or frozen turkey, 12–14 lbs.

10 cups stuffing (see recipe on page 137)

2 tablespoons butter

1 teaspoon rosemary

1 teaspoon thyme

Salt and pepper to taste

INSTRUCTIONS

Thaw and rinse bird thoroughly and pat dry. Place bird breast side up in a deep roasting pan and fill cavity with stuffing, being careful not to pack too tightly. Smooth neck skin over stuffing and tie legs together. Rub butter on turkey skin and sprinkle with rosemary, thyme, salt, and pepper. (If you use a meat thermometer, stick it into the center of a thigh without touching the bone.) Roast at 325 degrees for 4–4 $1/2$ hours, or time suggested for the weight of your turkey. Baste turkey every hour with the drippings from the roasting pan. Loosely cover turkey with foil for the last two hours of roasting. Start testing turkey for doneness an hour before roasting time is up. Let turkey stand 15–20 minutes before carving.

Number of portions depends on weight of turkey.

Mushroom and Red Wine Turkey Gravy

*Flavorful gravy made with turkey drippings
and a dash of red wine is the perfect accompaniment
to a roasted turkey dinner.*

INGREDIENTS

Turkey drippings from roasting pan

4 cups chicken broth

I can cream of mushroom soup

$1/4$ cup red wine

$1/2$ teaspoon salt

$1/2$ teaspoon pepper

Note: If thicker gravy is desired, add 1–2 tablespoons of whole-wheat flour.

INSTRUCTIONS

Combine all ingredients in a large pot over medium heat and bring to a boil. Lower heat and simmer for 5–10 minutes.

Makes twelve $1/2$-cup servings

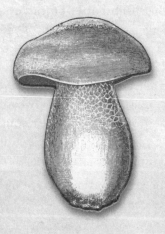

Tom's Turkey Stuffing

This classic stuffing made with whole-wheat bread
is a delicious and healthy way to stuff your bird.

INGREDIENTS

1 stick butter

1 cup onion, chopped

1 cup celery, chopped

1 large apple, chopped

1/2 cup raisins

1 teaspoon salt

1/2 cup walnuts, chopped

2 cups chicken broth or orange juice

6 cups whole-wheat bread, cubed

INSTRUCTIONS

Melt butter and sauté onions and celery in a large pan for 5 minutes or until tender. Add apples, raisins, salt, and walnuts, and sauté another 5 minutes. Add chicken broth or juice and heat to boiling. Place bread cubes in a large bowl and add sautéed mixture. Let it cool and stuff turkey.

Makes ten 1-cup servings

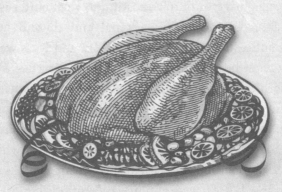

DAIRY

MILK

Use whole, organic milk. Half a cup of whole milk added to your cooked oatmeal or rice is a great way to add protein to your daily diet and also help to slow digestion. One-half cup of whole milk provides 4 grams of protein. You may even add $1/3$ cup of boiled custard (*see* recipe in Chapter 15) to your bread pudding or fruit if you like. Boiled custard is sweet and has a high protein content because it is made with whole milk and eggs.

Note: If you have high cholesterol or heart disease or are trying to decrease fat and cholesterol in your diet, substitute whole milk with 2-percent or fat-free milk. Two-percent milk has some fat and this will give you a creamy consistency with less fat.

BUTTER

Butter was an important part of the American Colonial diet and, when used in moderation, it can be beneficial to your health. It is important to have the freshest butter possible because you'll be using real butter to cook with, and you may want to use it as a condiment on your bread.

Never use margarine or butter substitutes. Real butter is rich in vitamin A, which is important for adrenal and thyroid health. Butter also contains antioxidants and vitamins D, E, and K, as well as lecithin, which promotes a healthy metabolism. The properties of butter help the body absorb calcium and help protect the teeth against decay. Fresh butter has also been found to protect against hardening of the arteries and cataracts. Use butter in moderation. Have no more than 2 teaspoons with a meal and only consume it in combination with whole grains.

In Colonial America, butter was churned in large crocks with wooden paddles. Making butter was a time-consuming, but necessary, task for colonial women. Now you can make a half-pound of delicious, fresh butter at home in about fifteen minutes using an electric mixer. Some store-bought butter is made from the pasteurized milk of cows that may have been treated with growth and milk-producing hormones. Even if you buy organic butter at the store, chances are it was made weeks earlier and is not as fresh as butter you can make at home. When you make your own butter, use organic cream from your local health food store.

INGREDIENTS

1 pint whole organic cream

salt (to taste)

INSTRUCTIONS

Pour cream into in a mixing bowl and mix on medium speed for about 8–10 minutes. The cream will turn into fluffy, stiff whipped cream. Keep mixing and the cream will start to turn grainy and pale yellow. It will soon look like fluffy, scrambled eggs. Keep mixing until it separates. The yellow butter granules will start sticking together in an unmistakable mass of butter and a watery milk-like liquid, known as buttermilk, will suddenly appear when the fats have separated and the butter is in a semi-solid state. When this happens, stop mixing because the process is finished. Remove the butter from the mixing bowl and form it into a ball in your hands, squeezing out any additional buttermilk water. (You can save the buttermilk for breadmaking if you desire.)

Rinse the ball under cold water for a moment and then squeeze it again. Repeat until the water runs clear.* Pat the butterball dry with a clean dishcloth to remove excess water and set it a small bowl. Stir in salt to taste, or keep it unsalted if you prefer. Leave the butter in the small bowl to harden, or store it in a butter crock or butter mold. Set it in the refrigerator to chill.

* It is important to rinse until you remove all the milky residue from the butterball. If you don't, your butter will quickly become rancid.

CHEESE

Cheese is a great source of protein, fat and calcium. Colonial housewives used to make cheese for the family using fresh milk. The milk would be heated in large pots over an open fire until warm, then they would add a tiny piece of a dried calf's stomach, known as rennin. After curds had formed, the cheese would be pressed and rubbed with salt to prevent mold and to help the hard cheese form a skin.

Cheese may be eaten on the Ben Franklin Diet, but only in combination with whole grains. Use natural cheeses such as cheddar, mozzarella, Gruyère, Parmesan, Jack, or Swiss and avoid processed cheeses like American. You can also eat soft cheeses on this diet, such as cream cheese and cottage cheese. Stilton (blue cheese) and Parmesan cheese were also popular in Colonial America. Parmesan cheese was one of Benjamin Franklin's favorites. He wrote in a letter to a friend, *"And for one I confess that if I could find in any Italian Travels a Receipt (recipe) for making Parmesan cheese it would give me more Satisfaction than a Transcript of any Inscription from any old Stone whatever."* In response, Franklin's friend sent him a recipe for making parmesan cheese.

Both hard and soft cheeses can be eaten on the Ben Franklin Diet, but not more than one ounce of cheese per meal, such as a slice on a piece of whole-grain bread or a tablespoon of soft cheese on whole-grain crackers.

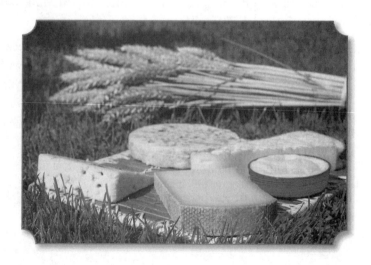

Colonial Garlic and Herb Cream Cheese

To make a delicious garlic and herb flavored variety of cheese, add the following herbs to an 8-ounce package of cream cheese.

INGREDIENTS

2 teaspoons minced garlic

1/4 teaspoon oregano

1/4 teaspoon black pepper

1/4 teaspoon parsley

1/4 teaspoon thyme

1/4 teaspoon sage

1/4 teaspoon paprika

1/4 teaspoon rosemary

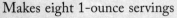

INSTRUCTIONS

Mix herbs into cream cheese until well blended. Enjoy with whole-wheat bread, homemade oatcakes, vegetable sticks, or whole-wheat crackers.

Makes eight 1-ounce servings

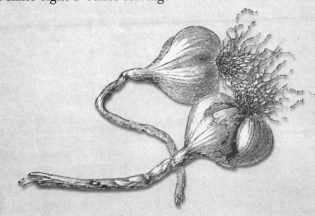

15

Sweet Fare

*B*y the late 1700s, sugar and molasses were common in Colonial America. Imported from the Caribbean islands, sugar was a valuable commodity, a barrel of brown sugar worth a set of chairs. While white sugar did exist in the colonial era, it was not common and was far more costly than the brown variety. Remaining true to their colonial heritage, most of the recipes in this section call for raw sugar.

The pies, puddings, and sweet dishes in this section are made with whole grains, ripe fruit, and wholesome ingredients. In other words, they are good for you. So don't be afraid to indulge occasionally and make a meal out of these sweet delights.

Note: If you have high cholesterol or heart disease or are trying to decrease fat and cholesterol in your diet, substitute whole milk with 2-percent or fat-free milk. Two-percent milk has some fat and this will give you a creamy consistency with less fat.

Boiled Vanilla Custard

Boiled custard was a colonial favorite. With a light vanilla flavor and smooth texture, this creamy custard turns the ordinary into the extraordinary. Each serving has about 6 grams of protein. This wholesome custard can be served over bread pudding, with fresh fruit, or all by itself as a meal. Thomas Tryon recommended eating custard and said, "Milk made boiling hot, and then thickened with eggs, is a brave substantial food of a friendly and mild nature and operation, agreeable to most or all people." *Boiled custard is a dessert that's good for you and can be enjoyed often.*

INGREDIENTS

2 cups whole milk

2 teaspoons cornstarch

2 eggs

3 tablespoons raw sugar

1 teaspoon vanilla extract

INSTRUCTIONS

Combine ¼ cup of milk with cornstarch and stir until dissolved. Add eggs to the milk/cornstarch mixture and whisk until smooth. Set aside. Combine 1¾ cups of milk and sugar in a heavy saucepan over medium heat and bring to a boil while stirring constantly to avoid scorching. Lower heat to a simmer and, in a steady stream, pour in the milk/egg/cornstarch mixture. Stir constantly for about 5 minutes until the mixture thickens to the consistency of heavy cream. Stir in vanilla. Remove from heat and pour into a jar. Serve hot over bread pudding, fresh fruit, or oatmeal in place of milk and sugar. Refrigerate unused custard.

Makes four 1-half-cup servings

Colonial Bread Pudding

*A serving of sweet, wholesome bread pudding makes
a great meal. Egg and milk add extra protein to this dish.
Try it for breakfast.*

INGREDIENTS

1 cup whole milk

1/4 cup brown sugar

1 egg

1/2 teaspoon vanilla extract

8 ounces whole-grain bread, cubed and weighed
(weigh bread on a scale because different breads
have different weights)

1/2 teaspoon ground cinnamon

1 tablespoon softened butter

INSTRUCTIONS

Preheat oven to 375 degrees. Combine milk, sugar, egg, and vanilla in a bowl and whisk until smooth. Add bread cubes to milk mixture. Stir until all bread pieces are coated. Add cinnamon and softened butter and stir until mixed. Grease a loaf pan with butter and press mixture into it. Bake for 40 minutes or until knife inserted in center comes out clean. Serve warm with a small dollop of whipped cream (optional) or a small amount of boiled vanilla custard.

Makes four 1-cup servings

Brown Rice Pudding

*A serving of creamy rice pudding is a great way to eat
your grains at any meal. This colonial pudding is made
with whole milk, brown rice, raisins and a bit of sugar
and spice. Thomas Tryon said of this dish,* "Rice Puddings
both plain and made of Fruit, which for the most part
are a pleasant sort of food, easie of digestion, and may
be freely eaten." *While this old-fashioned pudding takes
two hours to cook, it's well worth the wait.*

INGREDIENTS

2 cups whole milk

1/4 cup uncooked brown rice

2 tablespoons raw sugar

1/4 teaspoon ground nutmeg

1/4 cup raisins (optional)

INSTRUCTIONS

Combine milk, rice, sugar, and nutmeg in a 1-quart glass mason
jar and stir until blended. The jar will be halfway full. Cover the
top of the jar tightly with a piece of aluminum foil. Place the
mason jar in a large soup pot and fill the pot with enough water
to halfway immerse the mason jar. Bring the water to a boil over
medium heat and let it boil uncovered for two hours. Check the
pot after one hour and add more water as needed to ensure that
the boiling water remains at the same level as the pudding inside
the mason jar. When cooked, take the jar out of the pot and
remove the foil. Stir in raisins. As the pudding cools down, it will
thicken. Serve the pudding warm.

Makes two 1-cup servings

Gingersnaps

Gingersnap cookies are just as popular today as they were in Colonial America. Besides being delicious, this authentic recipe is good for you. Made with molasses and whole-wheat flour, these tasty little cookies are a healthy treat you can enjoy anytime.

INGREDIENTS

1 cup molasses

$1/4$ cup vegetable shortening

1 teaspoon baking soda

$1/8$ teaspoon salt

2 teaspoons ground ginger

$13/4$ cups whole-wheat flour

INSTRUCTIONS

Preheat oven to 400 degrees. Combine the molasses and shortening in a saucepan over medium heat and bring to a boil. Stir in baking soda, salt, and ginger. Mixture will become foamy and lighter in color. Remove from heat and let it cool. Transfer mixture to a bowl and add the flour, stirring until well blended. Drop dough in rounded teaspoons onto an ungreased cookie sheet and bake for 6 minutes.

Makes 3 dozen cookies; 6 cookies make a $1/2$-cup serving

Harvest Pumpkin Pie

This light and fluffy pumpkin pie is a delicious treat you can enjoy year-round. Brown sugar, maple syrup, and extra cinnamon give this pie a sweet and spicy flavor like no other.

INGREDIENTS FOR FILLING

15 oz. cooked pumpkin (homemade or canned)

$1/2$ cup brown sugar

$1/2$ cup whole milk

3 eggs

$1/4$ cup pure maple syrup

1 tablespoon dark rum

2 teaspoons ground cinnamon

$1/2$ teaspoon ground nutmeg

$1/2$ teaspoon ground cloves

$1/2$ teaspoon ground ginger

$1/4$ teaspoon sea salt

HOW TO COOK A PUMPKIN

Choose a small, firm *pie* pumpkin about the size of a soccer ball. Cut the pumpkin in half and scrape out all seeds and stringy pulp. Place the two pumpkin halves on a greased cookie sheet and bake at 300 degrees for 1 hour. When you remove the pumpkin halves, the flesh should be soft enough to scrape it from the skin. Place the cooked pumpkin in a bowl and mash it with an electric mixer or a potato masher. Proceed with the recipe as follows.

INSTRUCTIONS

Preheat oven to 375 degrees. Combine all ingredients in a large bowl and mix until well blended. Set aside while you make the pie crust.

INGREDIENTS FOR A SWEET WHOLE WHEAT PIE CRUST

$1^1/_2$ cups whole-wheat flour

2 tablespoons brown sugar

$^1/_2$ teaspoon salt

$^1/_3$ cup butter (6 tablespoons)

7–8 tablespoons ice water

INSTRUCTIONS FOR A SWEET WHOLE WHEAT PIE CRUST

Combine flour, sugar, and salt in a bowl. Cut butter into small pieces and add it to the flour. Using your fingers, crush the butter pieces into the flour mixture. Add 7 tablespoons ice water and continue mixing the flour with your hands. Form it into a ball. Add another tablespoon of water if the dough seems too dry to work with. Place the dough ball on a floured surface and roll it out flat, to about $^1/_8$ inch thick.

Place the dough in a greased 9" deep-dish pie plate and press it into shape. Prick the bottom of the crust with a fork, then bake it for 10 minutes at 375 to brown it. Pour the pumpkin mix into the pie shell and bake for 60 minutes or until knife inserted in center of pie comes out clean. Serve warm or room temperature.

Makes six 1-cup servings, or one deep-dish pie

Cranberry Tarts

Benjamin Franklin enjoyed cranberries so much that he had his wife Deborah ship them over to England during his extended stay there. His friends knew how much he liked them as well. Jonathan Williams wrote in a letter to Franklin, "I have lately received some Cranberrys from Boston. I will pick out enough to make you a few Cranberry Tarts."

This recipe is for a batch of delicious miniature cranberry tarts made with whole wheat and fruit. These tarts can be eaten as a snack or warmed and eaten for breakfast.

INGREDIENTS FOR CRANBERRY FILLING

$1/2$ cup dried cranberries

$1/2$ cup apple juice

$1/4$ cup raw sugar

$1/4$ cup chopped dates

3 tablespoons lemon juice

1 teaspoon whole-wheat flour

INSTRUCTIONS TO MAKE FILLING

Combine all ingredients in a saucepan and bring to a boil over medium heat with constant stirring. Cook for 5–7 minutes until liquid looks like thick syrup. Remove from heat and set aside.

INGREDIENTS FOR CRUST

$1^1/2$ cups whole-wheat flour

$1/3$ cup butter (6 tablespoons)

7–8 tablespoons ice water

2 tablespoons brown sugar

$1/2$ teaspoon salt

INSTRUCTIONS TO MAKE CRUST

Preheat the oven to 400 degrees. Combine flour, sugar and salt in a bowl. Cut butter into small pieces and add it to flour. Using your fingers, crush the butter pieces into the flour mixture. Add 7 tablespoons ice water and continue mixing the flour with your hands. Form it into a ball. Add another tablespoon of water if the dough seems too dry to work with. Place the dough ball on a floured surface and roll it out flat (about 1/8-inch thick). Cut the dough into 3 x 3 inch squares. Form the dough scraps into a new ball and roll flat to make more squares.

Once your squares are cut, place 1 tablespoon of cranberry filling in the center of each. Fold the square into a triangle over the filling and pinch the edges of the dough closed with your fingers, careful not to let the filling leak out the sides. Prick the edges of each triangle with the tines of a fork to reinforce the seal. Cut two 1/2-inch slits in to top of each tart. Brush tarts with milk and sprinkle a small amount of raw sugar on top of each. Place tarts on a greased cookie sheet and bake for 20 minutes. Remove from oven and serve hot.

Makes eight 2ounce servings (about 1/2-cup in volume each)

Note: Boiled custard is a perfect accompaniment to these sweet and sour tarts. Pour a little over the top.

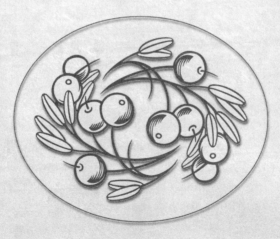

Colonial Green Apple and Pear Pie

The combination of tart, green apples and sweet pears makes a delicious fruit pie. Thomas Tryon recommended eating both apple and pear pies and wrote in his 1691 cookbook, "Apple Pies made with Fruit, that is neither too green or unripe, not too cold or far spent, are a very good Food, especially for young People; they afford a good nourishment, and are friendly to Nature . . . Pear Pies being full, and ripe, makes a fine, gentle, friendly Food of easie Concoction."

With very little sugar and plenty of whole-wheat goodness, this apple and pear pie can be enjoyed as dessert or a meal.

INGREDIENTS

6 medium ripe green apples

2 ripe pears (or substitute with 1 cup canned and drained pears)

1/4 cup brown sugar

1/4 cup whole-wheat flour

1 teaspoon ground cinnamon

1/2 teaspoon ground nutmeg

Double pie crust (see below)

1 tablespoon butter

INSTRUCTIONS

Preheat oven to 350 degrees. Peel, core and cut apples and pears into very thin slices (this is the key to getting a firm, yet cooked texture). In a large bowl, combine apple slices, sugar, flour, cinnamon, and nutmeg, and toss until evenly mixed. Transfer apples into a pie shell. Cut butter into small pieces and place on top of the apple filling. Cover apples with the second pie crust and pinch both crusts together at the edges. Cut a 1 inch slit in the top crust. Bake for 40–45 minutes.

INGREDIENTS FOR A DOUBLE PIE CRUST

2 cups whole-wheat flour

2 tablespoons brown sugar

1 teaspoon salt

$^3/_4$ cup vegetable shortening

5–6 tablespoons ice water

INSTRUCTIONS FOR A DOUBLE PIE CRUST

Combine flour, sugar, and salt in a bowl and stir. Add shortening to mixture. Using your fingers, crush the shortening into the flour mixture. Add 5 tablespoons ice water and continue mixing with your hands. Form dough into a ball. Add another tablespoon of water if the dough seems too dry to work with.

Divide the dough into two equal pieces and place balls on a floured surface. Roll each ball out flat (about $^1/_8$-inch thick). Place one crust in a greased pie dish and press into shape. Set the other crust aside until you've added the filling.

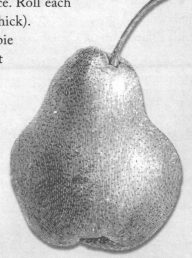

Makes six 1-cup servings, or one deep-dish pie.

Apple Brown Betty

This is a simple colonial dish made with apples, bread, and mouth-watering cinnamon. Reminiscent of apple pie, this recipe is a great way to turn your unused bread slices into a delicious treat.

INGREDIENTS

4 large apples

2 cups bread, cubed

$1/2$ cup raw sugar

$1/4$ cup melted butter

2 teaspoons cinnamon

$1/2$ cup water

INSTRUCTIONS

Preheat oven to 350 degrees. Peel, core, and slice apples. Combine apples, bread crumbs, sugar, melted butter, and cinnamon, and toss until evenly mixed. Place mixture in a greased baking dish and pour the water over the top. Bake for 45 minutes. Serve warm with Boiled Vanilla Custard over the top.

Makes four 1-cup servings

Spiced Apples

This easy-to-make treat can be enjoyed anytime.

INGREDIENTS

2 apples, peeled and diced

1 teaspoon ground cinnamon

1 teaspoon raw sugar

INSTRUCTIONS

Combine all ingredients in a bowl and toss until mixed. Enjoy them immediately or warm the dish in the oven until apples are tender.

Makes two 1-cup servings.

VARIATION

Broken raw walnut pieces in the mix add a nice crunch and are very healthy.

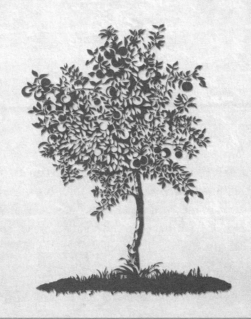

Raisin and Prune Bread Pudding

This recipe was adapted from Thomas Tryon's vegetarian cookbook published in 1691. "Take Raisins, Currans and a few Pruens, boil them in good Water, when near done thicken it with white Bread, adding Spice, Sugar, Butter and Salt; this is a rich Pottage, affording a great nourishment, and therefore it must be eaten the more sparingly."
A combination of raisins, prunes, spices, and bread makes a delicious treat to enjoy anytime.

INGREDIENTS

1 cup whole-grain bread, cubed

1/4 cup raisins

1/4 cup prunes

1 cup water

1 tablespoon butter

2 teaspoons raw sugar

1/2 teaspoon cinnamon

Pinch of ground cloves

Pinch of salt

INSTRUCTIONS

Combine raisins, prunes, and water in a saucepan and bring to a boil over medium heat. Boil for five minutes to soften fruit. Reduce heat to simmer and add butter, sugar, cinnamon, cloves, and salt. Remove from heat and add cubed bread, stirring and smashing until the mixture is blended. Serve hot.

Makes two 1/2-cup servings

Colonial Peach Cobbler

*Peach cobbler was a popular dessert in Colonial America. Sweet,
seasonal peaches and a dash of dark rum make this rustic dish
irresistible. Whether you serve it for dessert or enjoy it for
breakfast, cobbler is a fantastic way to enjoy ripe, fresh peaches.*

INGREDIENTS

6 ripe peaches, pitted and sliced thin
(leave unpeeled for a rustic cobbler)

1 cup whole-wheat flour, plus $1/4$ cup

$1/2$ cup walnuts, chopped

$1/4$ cup butter, softened

$1/2$ cup raw sugar plus 1 tablespoon

1 tablespoon dark rum

2 eggs

1 teaspoon baking soda

1 teaspoon cinnamon

$1/2$ teaspoon salt

INSTRUCTIONS

Preheat the oven to 350 degrees. Place peach slices in a large bowl.
Add $1/4$ cup flour and walnuts and toss until coated. Set aside.
In another bowl combine butter, sugar, rum, and eggs, and stir
until blended. Add flour, baking soda, cinnamon, and salt, and
stir until smooth. Batter will be thick. Flour and grease a loaf pan
and spread half of the batter in the bottom. Layer the peach slices
and walnut mixture on the batter. Take the remaining batter and
carefully spread it over the layer of peaches. Sprinkle 1 tablespoon
of raw sugar on top of the batter and place the pan in the oven.
Bake for 30 minutes. Slice cobbler and serve warm.

Makes eight 1-cup servings

Strawberry Maple Pie

Strawberry pie is a tasty way to enjoy strawberries while they're fresh and in-season. This recipe for strawberry pie is even sweeter with a little bit of maple syrup and brown sugar.

INGREDIENTS

1 tablespoon pure maple syrup

1/4 cup raw sugar

Juice of half a lemon

4 cups sliced fresh strawberries

1 unbaked pie shell

INSTRUCTIONS

Combine maple syrup, sugar, and the juice of half a lemon in a small saucepan over low heat and stir until sugar is dissolved. Pour the sugar mixture over the strawberries and toss gently until strawberries are coated. Refrigerate until cool.

INGREDIENTS/INSTRUCTIONS FOR CRUST

See the recipe for Harvest Pumpkin Pie earlier in this chapter for instructions on making a sweet whole-wheat pie crust.

INSTRUCTIONS TO BAKE PIE

Preheat oven to 400 degrees. Prick the bottom of the unbaked pie shell with a fork, place in preheated oven and bake for 10 minutes or until crust is golden. Remove shell from oven and allow to cool to room temperature. Pour strawberries into pie shell and refrigerate. Cut into slices and serve with a little whipped cream on top.

Makes six 1-cup servings, or one deep-dish pie

16

Sweeteners, Spices, and Condiments

*Y*ou may use raw sugar, honey, or maple syrup sparingly, no more than two teaspoons of sweetener per meal. Salt is allowed, but it should also be used sparingly. Instead of salt, experiment with spices and condiments, such as cinnamon, garlic, ginger, mustard, or pepper.

SWEETENERS

Some of the recipes in this book call for raw or unrefined sugar, which is the type of sugar that was available in eighteenth-century America. While white, refined sugar was being produced at the time, it was expensive and hard to come by. All sugar should be used sparingly in the diet, but raw sugar is *slightly* more beneficial to the body than refined white sugar, which has *no* nutritional value. Raw sugar, also called *turbinado* sugar, is derived from the juice of sugar cane, and comes in larger, golden crystals. It contains nutrients and minerals, including calcium, iron, magnesium, phosphorus, and potassium. Raw sugar is not the same as *brown sugar,* which is often refined, processed sugar that has had molasses added to it. You can buy raw, unrefined sugar at your local health food store, and some grocery stores also carry a brand called *Sugar in the Raw.* You can use raw sugar in baking and get the same results as with refined sugar. A teaspoon or two of raw sugar can be used to sweeten your oatmeal or coffee, but practice temperance. You can use brown sugar on the Ben Franklin Diet instead of raw sugar, but make sure that it is natural, pure cane brown sugar.

Remember, all sugars are simple carbohydrates that result in spikes of insulin levels and speeded-up digestion. If you want to lose weight and slow your digestion, cut out sugar wherever you can.

Honey may be used as a sweetener in place of sugar, but again, only in very small amounts, no more than 2 teaspoons per meal. *"Bread and honey is pleasant and wholesome eating,"* Franklin wrote in' 1765. *"'Tis a sweet that does not hurt the teeth. How many fine sets might be saved; and what an infinite quantity of tooth ache avoided!"*

Note: Do not consume drinks or products made with high-fructose corn syrup or artificial sweeteners.

EAST INDIES SPICES

By the end of the eighteenth century, England had become the center of the world spice trade. The colonists in America used spices in their cooking and relied on imported spices from the motherland. Colonial American cooking included the use of many spices and goods imported from the East Indies, which were sent to the colonies by ship. Some of the most popular imports were pepper, cinnamon, cloves, ginger root, and nutmeg. These spices, featured prominently in colonial cooking, will give your meals an authentic and delicious flavor.

To get the maximum health benefits and flavor from your spices, it is recommended that you buy them in small quantities. Because spices are seeds and roots that have been dried, they will lose their flavor over time, some in as little as three months. While pre-ground spices will suffice, whole spices are more aromatic because the oils haven't fully dissipated. It is recommended that you grind the spices yourself to experience the maximum flavor. Use either a small electric coffee grinder or a mortar and pestle, or place the spices in a heavy plastic bag and crush them into a powder with a rolling pin. Some spices, such as nutmeg and cinnamon, should be grated using a small metal grater. Grate enough spices for immediate use and store your unused spices in closed bottles or containers. Spices keep best in a cool, dry place out of direct sunlight.

COLONIAL PANTRY LIST FOR SPICES AND HERBS

These are some of the spices you will commonly find in Colonial American cooking and their benefits.

NAME	BENEFITS
Allspice	Helps maintain proper digestion, prevents intestinal gas and can relieve joint pain
Black Pepper	Helps maintain proper digestion and helps with weight loss by breaking down fat cells, prevents intestinal gas, a good antioxidant, relieves sinusitis and nasal congestion, and can relieve joint pain
Cayenne Pepper	Helps reduce psoriasis and inflammation in asthma, joints, and sinuses, contains natural antibiotic and anti-viral properties and works as a natural pain reliever, also increases circulation in the body and prevents blood clots.
Cinnamon	Reduces blood-sugar levels, lowers cholesterol, aids digestion, treats diarrhea, relieves pain, boosts memory, treats tooth pain, eases headaches
Cloves	Anti-inflammatory, used for treating pain, including tooth-aches, used as an aphrodisiac, and to prevent blood clots
Ginger	Treats nausea, helps maintain proper digestion, can relieve diarrhea, joint pain, and menstrual cramps, used as an aphrodisiac
Nutmeg	Increases blood circulation, promotes sleep, relieves pain, relieves congestion, and can help boost concentration, used as aphrodisiac
Rosemary	Calms nerves, relaxes muscles, improves circulation, aids digestion, used to relieve headaches
Sage	Has anti-fungal properties, used to treat skin wounds, improves memory, sharpens senses
Thyme	Has anti-bacterial properties, used as anti-inflammatory, relieves menstrual cramps, used as a natural food preservative
Vanilla	Used to calm a queasy stomach and reduce anxiety, an antioxidant containing small amounts of B vitamins and minerals

Colonial Vanilla Rum Extract

The finest vanilla extracts in the world are made from dried vanilla beans preserved in alcohol. The oils from the beans are drawn out by the alcohol and create an aromatic infusion. Cheap, imitation vanilla flavorings are made from wood pulp, coal tar, sassafras, and chemicals. It's fun and easy to make your own genuine colonial vanilla extract for use in recipes calling for the delightful flavor of vanilla.

INGREDIENTS

1 whole vanilla bean

$1/2$ cup dark rum

INSTRUCTIONS

Cut the vanilla bean into pieces and place it in a mason jar with the rum. Close the jar and let it sit in a cool, dark place for two weeks, giving it a gentle shake every few days. After two weeks, the vanilla extract is ready to use. Discard the pieces of vanilla bean and transfer the extract to a glass bottle tinted amber or blue. Store the bottle in a cool, dark place.

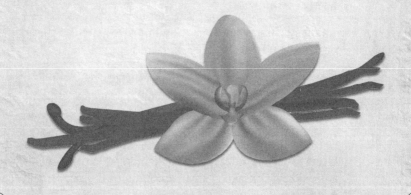

THE BENEFITS OF GINGER

When seafaring colonists ate their gingerbread (*see* Gingerbread recipe in Chapter 12), they were availing themselves of one of nature's most powerful healing herbs. Besides handling nausea, ginger has other health benefits—it helps blood circulation and naturally eases joint and muscle pain. In one clinical study, a group of test subjects with rheumatoid arthritis who had failed to get relief from conventional drugs took five grams of fresh ginger daily and all reported substantial improvements, including reduced pain, greater joint mobility, and decreased swelling and stiffness. Ginger can help break fevers and is also a very effective expectorant that helps to get rid of phlegm.

While dried ginger powder is available in the spice aisle, fresh grated ginger is the best, especially the organic variety, which is stronger. Fresh ginger is available at most grocery stores for pennies. To grate it, remove the outer skin and grate with a fine cheese grater. Grate only as much as you need and store the unused ginger in a bag or covered container in the refrigerator. It keeps for up to a week.

Alternatively, you can treat it as they do in Asia. Cut off as much as you want for a single serving, remove the thin peel with the side of a spoon, then slice the peeled section, pound the slices with the blunt end of a knife to release the juices, and chop to put into tea or similar. Drinking the hot beverage, then eating the ginger bits will make your body very happy—it will say, *Thank you, thank you*

Mustard

Mustard is a spicy condiment you can enjoy with your homemade bread. A turkey sandwich spiced with homemade mustard is a delight to the taste buds. Making your own mustard is fast and easy. There are three types of mustard seeds—black, brown, and yellow. The black seeds are the spiciest and are used in Indian cooking. The brown seeds are pungent and medium in spiciness and are used to make Dijon mustard. The yellow seeds are mild and are used to make American yellow mustard. You can purchase whole mustard seeds at some ethnic grocery stores or through the suppliers listed in Resources in the back of this book. Whichever types of mustard seed you choose, have fun creating your own unique blends.

Basic Mustard Recipe

You will need a small mortar and pestle to grind your mustard seeds into powder. These are available at cooking supply stores or through the suppliers in Resources in the back of the book.

INGREDIENTS

$1/2$ cup ground mustard seeds (brown or yellow)
or pre-ground yellow mustard powder

$1/4$ cup water

2 tablespoons red wine vinegar

I teaspoon sea salt

INSTRUCTIONS

Add water and vinegar to ground mustard seeds. Stir until well blended. Store in a jar in the refrigerator.

VARIATIONS:

• Try adding ingredients, such as a teaspoon of crushed garlic, horseradish, or other herbs and spices.

• Try using ale, champagne, or honey, instead of vinegar.

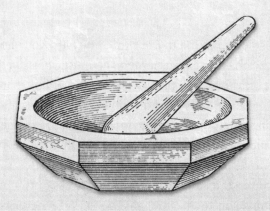

17

Drinks

*W*hile water is the best thing you can drink, you may drink tea and coffee on the Ben Franklin Diet as long as you do so in moderation. If you are sensitive to caffeine, drink decaffeinated coffee or tea, or delete it entirely from your diet.

WHITE PINE NEEDLE TEA

When the colonists first came to America, they soon ran out of coffee and tea from England. But much to their delight, they discovered that pine needles could be brewed to produce a hot beverage much like tea. Benjamin Franklin found pine needle tea delicious and said, "*...for tea, we have sage and bawm in our gardens, the young leaves of the sweet white hickory or walnut, and, above all, the buds of our pine, infinitely preferable to any tea from the Indies.*" With an abundant supply of pine needles, it was easy for colonists to make their own tea. Besides having a great, tangy taste, one cup of pine needle tea has five times more vitamin C than a whole lemon or an entire glass of orange juice. That's more than 400 milligrams per cup. Vitamin C is beneficial to boosting the immune system and can help improve cardiovascular system functions. Pine needle tea is also rich in vitamin A, which is needed for healthy vision, hair and skin regeneration, and red blood cell production.

How to Make White Pine Needle Tea

Before you begin, it is very important that you use a field guide to properly identify the white pine, as some species of pine trees are not suitable for making tea and can be toxic. Once you've identified a white pine tree (*Pinus strobus*), recognizable by its five-needle bundles, pick a handful of its fresh, green, pine needles. You will need enough to fill half a cup. Wash the needles under water to remove any dirt or debris. Snip off the brown ends with scissors, then cut the needles into pieces about one inch long. Measure out half a cup of needles. Bring 2 pints of water to a boil in a pan and add the pine needles. Cover the pan and lower the heat to simmer. After 20 minutes, remove from heat. The liquid will be a pale reddish/orange color. Strain out the pine needle pieces and serve hot. Add a teaspoon of honey or raw sugar if you like.

Portion size: 4 one-cup servings

Warning: Pregnant women should never drink pine needle tea as some species of pine contain toxic substances that can harm the fetus.

ADDITIONAL DRINK RECIPES

The following are recipes for some of the most popular drinks in colonial times. Be aware that these recipes are for occasional use only and should not be part of your regular diet as they have a high sugar content.

Benjamin Franklin's Spiced Milk Punch

Although Franklin wasn't a big drinker of alcoholic punch, he occasionally indulged in spirits. In a letter to his friend James Bowden in 1763, Franklin shared his recipe for spiced milk punch. This recipe has been altered to make a 32 oz. pitcher, perfect for a small gathering or party.

INGREDIENTS

6 lemons (or enough to squeeze 4 ounces of fresh lemon juice)

12 ounces brandy

8 ounces water

6 ounces whole milk

4 ounces refined sugar

1 teaspoon grated nutmeg

INSTRUCTIONS

Remove rinds from the lemons and let them soak overnight in the brandy . Squeeze all the juice from the lemons and refrigerate until you're ready to use it. The next day, remove the lemon rinds from the brandy and place them in a large pot. Add the water, milk, lemon juice, sugar, and nutmeg. Bring mixture to a boil over medium heat while stirring to avoid scalding. When the sugar is dissolved, remove from heat and stir. Let mixture sit undisturbed for 2 hours. To serve, strain the mixture through a cheesecloth or fine sieve until it is clear and place it in a punch bowl.

Makes eight 1-half-cup servings

VARIATION

To make a delicious non-alcoholic version, replace the brandy with apple cider.

Colonial Ginger Root Beer

A recipe for the truly adventurous. This sweet and spicy brew was popular among the colonists. Although this type of non-alcoholic ale is the basis for modern-day root beer and ginger ale, it tastes nothing like the commercially produced products on the shelves of the supermarket. In colonial times, root beer was flavored primarily with such roots as ginger or sassafras. If you want to make plain ginger ale, delete the sassafras from the recipe.

Note: Ginger root beer needs to ferment for 24 hours, but it's worth the wait.

INGREDIENTS

1 gallon purified water

4 ounces fresh ginger root, sliced

2 tablespoons dried sassafras bark

$1/4$ teaspoon ground cloves

$1/4$ teaspoon nutmeg

2 teaspoons yeast

1 lemon

1 cup raw sugar

INSTRUCTIONS

Boil $1/2$ gallon of water in a large pot. Add sliced fresh ginger, sassafras bark, cloves, and nutmeg to the boiling water. Cover the pot and simmer for fifteen minutes. Remove from heat and stir in the yeast until dissolved. Extract the juice from the lemon and add it to the mixture. Pour the mixture into a large plastic bottle, cap it, and let it ferment in a warm place for 24 hours. The next day, combine the sugar with $^1/_2$ cup hot water and stir until dissolved. Pour the liquid mixture into a clean bottle, straining out the spices as you do so, then add the sugar mixture and the rest of the water. Pour ginger root beer into two empty 2-liter plastic soda bottles and store in the refrigerator.

Makes sixteen 1-cup servings

Note: The reason to store your homemade ginger root beer in plastic instead of glass is that if the bottles get accidentally left out and they warm up, the fermentation process will start again and that could shatter glass.

VARIATION

To make your own root beer and ginger ale with a contemporary taste, you can buy all-natural flavor syrups and empty plastic bottles. (*See* list of suppliers in the Resources section in back.)

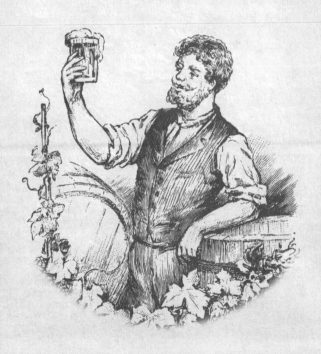

Spiced Apple Cider

A cup of delicious apple cider can be served hot or cold.
Cinnamon and cloves create a spicy, aromatic blend,
and a touch of raw sugar gives it a sweeter taste.

INGREDIENTS

$1/2$ gallon unfiltered organic apple juice

1 cinnamon stick

10 whole cloves

$1/4$ cup raw sugar

INSTRUCTIONS

Pour apple juice into a large pot and bring to a boil. Add cinnamon and cloves, reduce heat, cover pot and simmer for 30 minutes. Remove from heat and strain out cinnamon and cloves. Stir in sugar until dissolved.

Makes eight 1-cup servings

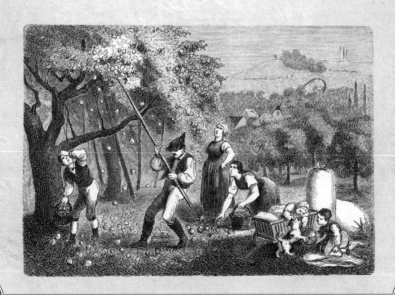

18

Sample Meal Plans

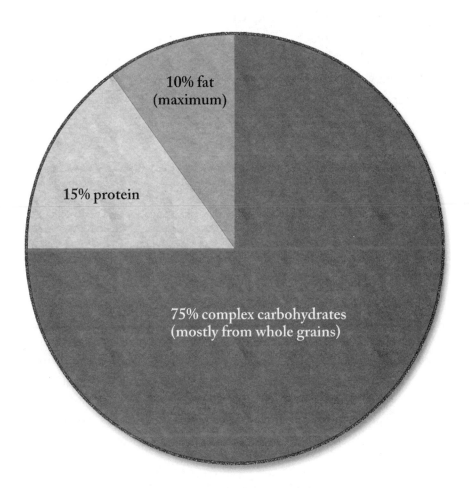

THE 75-15-10 FORMULA. This pie chart shows the proper proportions of whole grains, vegetables, protein, and fats, allowable per day. It gives you a good visual on the percentages of food types allowed per day on the diet.

There is a basic formula that makes up the Ben Franklin Diet that can be called the *75-15-10*, meaning that 75 percent of what you eat should be complex carbohydrates, around 15 percent should be protein, and a maximum of 10 percent fat. Use the 75-15-10 formula as a guideline to keep your meals balanced.

SAMPLE MEAL PLAN

Recipes from the book have been used to create samples of one-pint meals with a high proportion of whole grains. Your daily food allowance should be 75 percent complex carbohydrates, mainly in the form of whole grains. This translates to 3 pints, or 6 cups, of cooked whole grains, fresh vegetables, and small portions of in-season fruit per day. The remainder of your daily intake is a combination of small amounts of protein, dairy, and fat.

A NOTE ABOUT THE
SAMPLE MEAL PLAN

In the sample meal plan that follows, you will see suggestions for eating things like pumpkin pie; vanilla custard; peach cobbler; and turkey with gravy, stuffing, and all the trimmings as part of your diet. Yes, these delectable dishes are part of the Ben Franklin Diet, but only if you make them *yourself*, following the recipes in the cookbook section of this book, colonial-style recipes that are made with wholesome, healthy ingredients. Be aware, however, that you will *not* get the same health benefits and weight-loss results if you eat storebought pumpkin pie or peach cobbler typically made with white flour, refined sugar, and high-fructose corn syrup.

NINE DAYS OF THE BEN FRANKLIN DIET

DAY ONE

Breakfast
$1^1/_2$ cup Oatmeal with $^1/_2$ cup milk sweetened with
2 teaspoons of raw sugar or maple syrup and
1 teaspoon of butter
1 apple

Lunch
Turkey Sandwich made with two 4-ounce slices
of whole-grain bread and 3 ounces of turkey
with mustard and lettuce

Dinner
1 cup Pennsylvania Dutch Potato Soup and 4 ounces whole-
grain bread with 2 teaspoons butter or 1 ounce cheese

Snacks
6 Oatcakes with 1 ounce cheese, $^1/_4$ cup almonds,
and $^3/_4$ cup in-season berries

DAY TWO

Breakfast
$1^1/_2$ cup serving of Colonial Bread Pudding served hot
with $^1/_2$ cup Boiled Vanilla Custard

Lunch
2 Benjamin Franklin Meal-Replacement Bars

Dinner
2 cups Corn Chowder with chicken and 1 cup of raw
spinach with oil and vinegar dressing

Snacks
Two apples and $^1/_4$ cup almonds

DAY THREE

Breakfast
1 cup Hasty Pudding with 2 teaspoons butter,
2 teaspoons raw sugar, and a fresh pear

Lunch
1 cup Spicy Pumpkin Soup and a 5-ounce piece of
whole-grain rye bread with 2 teaspoons butter

Dinner
3 ounce Fish Fillet and $1^{1}/_{2}$ cups Brown Rice,
steamed

Snacks
4-ounce slice of whole-grain bread and a 4-ounce
piece of Buttermilk Carrot Loaf

DAY FOUR

Breakfast
$1^{1}/_{2}$ cups Oatmeal with $^{1}/_{2}$ cup milk and
2 teaspoons raw sugar

Lunch
1 cup Tavern Stew and 5 ounces whole-grain bread
with 2 teaspoons butter

Dinner
2 cups Baked Turkey Hotpot

Snacks
1 Benjamin Franklin Meal-Replacement Bar
and 1 cup chopped raw vegetables

DAY FIVE

Breakfast
Two 5-ounce pieces toasted whole-grain bread with
2 teaspoons butter and 2 teaspoons honey

Lunch
Tuna Sandwich made with 3 ounces tuna on whole-
grain bread with lettuce and tomato

Dinner
2 cups cooked Brown Rice with soy sauce
and fresh grated ginger

Snacks
2 Cranberry Tarts and 1 cup chopped carrots
and celery

DAY SIX

Breakfast
4-ounce slice of Colonial Gingerbread and 1 cup of
Oatmeal with $1/4$ cup milk and 2 teaspoons raw sugar

Lunch
5-ounce slice Colonial Buttermilk Bread
and 1 cup Onion and Ale Soup

Dinner
1 cup Tavern Stew and a 4-ounce chunk of Benjamin
Franklin's Maize and Whole Wheat Cornbread

Snacks
1 Benjamin Franklin Meal-Replacement Bar
and 1 cup blueberries

DAY SEVEN

Breakfast
2 Benjamin Franklin Meal-Replacement Bars

Lunch
1 cup Colonial Corn Chowder
and 5 ounces Sally Lunn Bread with 2 teaspoons
butter

Dinner
4 ounces Boston Brown Bread
and 3 ounces Grilled Chicken Breast

Snacks
1 slice of Harvest Pumpkin Pie,
$1/4$ cup nuts, and 1 apple

DAY EIGHT

Breakfast
1 slice of Harvest Pumpkin Pie
and 1 cup of Oatmeal with 2 teaspoons sugar
and 1 teaspoon butter

Lunch
2 cups Baked Turkey Hotpot

Dinner
1 cup Tom's Split Pea Porridge
and 1 cup Benjamin's Barley Casserole

Snacks
1 cup Brown Rice Pudding
and 1 cup Colonial Peach Cobbler

DAY NINE

Breakfast
2 Hoecakes with 2 teaspoons pure maple syrup
and 2 teaspoons butter, and 1 cup
Colonial Bread Pudding

Lunch
3 ounces Tom's Roasted Herb Turkey
with $1/2$ cup Mushroom & Red Wine Turkey Gravy
and 1 cup Tom's Turkey Stuffing

Dinner
1 cup Pennsylvania Dutch Potato Soup
and a 5-ounce piece of Colonial Chesterfield
Wheat Bread

Snacks
2 cups Popcorn and 4 ounces Blackberry Walnut
Bread

A Bill of Fare of Seventy-Five Noble Dishes of Excellent Food

THOMAS TRYON, 1691

As a teenager, Benjamin Franklin purchased a cookbook by an author named Thomas Tryon. The cookbook was titled *Wisdom's Dictates: or Aphorism's and Rules, Physical, Moral and Divine; For Preserving the Health of the Body and the Peace of the Mind, fit to be regarded and practiced by all that would enjoy the Blessings of the present and future World. A Bill of Fare of Seventy five Noble Dishes of Excellent Food, far exceeding those made of Fish and Flesh, which Banquet I present to the Sons of Wisdom, or such as shall decline that depraved Custom of Eating Flesh and Blood.*

Tryon's book is believed to be the first published vegetarian cookbook. Tryon advocated a diet without meat and gave instructions to prepare meals made of whole grains, vegetables, and dairy products. Tryon believed that a person could achieve health, happiness, and long life by eating grain, plants, and dairy, including eggs.

Always looking for ways to save money, Franklin implemented Tryon's vegetarian diet and, simply by cutting meat out of his diet, he was able to save over half the wages he earned as his brother's assistant at the print shop. In fact, he saved so much money that he was able to purchase more books and move out of his brother's house into lodgings of his own.

Franklin wrote in his autobiography, *"I made my self acquainted with Tryon's Manner of preparing some of his Dishes, such as Boiling Potatoes, or Rice, making Hasty Pudding, & a few others. I presently found that I could save half what he [Franklin's brother] paid me. This was an additional Fund*

for buying Books. But I had another Advantage in it. My Brother and the
rest going from the Printing House to their Meals, I remain'd there alone,
and dispatching presently my light Repast, (which often was no more than a
Bisket or a Slice of Bread, a Handful of Raisins or a Tart from the Pastry
Cook's, and a Glass of Water) had the rest of the Time till their Return, for
Study, in which I made the greatest Progress from that Greater Clearness of
Head & quicker Apprehension which usually attend Temperance in Eating
and Drinking."

As a young man, Franklin learned the value of eating light, a discovery
that served as the foundation of his lifelong dining habits. Eating bread
and oatmeal and drinking water were the top recommendations in
Thomas Tryon's book. Specifically, Tryon said of the regimen, *"Bread and*
water hath the first place of all foods, and are the foundation of dry moist
nourishment. Take oatmeal and make it into a gruel and put bread into it and
season it with salt. This and bread and a glass of water, a man may live very
well . . . Let your Food be simple, and Drinks innocent and learn of Wisdom
and Experience how to prepare them aright."

Although Benjamin Franklin later resumed eating small amounts of
fish, fowl, and red meat, the majority of his diet consisted of whole grains.
By experimentation, he observed that eating little or no meat kept his
head clear and increased his ability to absorb knowledge when studying.

Following is Thomas Tryon's vegetarian cookbook and instructions to
make seventy-five vegetarian dishes. You will find that the food is indeed
simple and easy to prepare.

A BILL OF FARE OF SEVENTY-FIVE NOBLE DISHES
OF EXCELLENT FOOD (THOMAS TRYON)

Of several Excellent Dishes of Food, easily procured without Flesh and
Blood, or the Dying growns [groans] of God's innocent and harmless
creatures, which do as far exceed those made of Flesh and Fish, as the
Light doth Darkness, or the Day the Night, and will satisfie all the wants
of Nature to the biggest Degree; which Banquet I present to the Sons of
Wisdom, and to all such as shall obtain that happy Condition, as to decline
that depraved Custom of killing and Eating their Fellow Creatures, and

whose desire is to live according to the innocent Law of Nature, and do unto all Creatures as they would be done unto; for the highest degree of Sanctity and Religion, is to imitate God, who is the Maker and Preserver of all things: Consider also, that thy Life is near and dear to thee, that like is to be understood of all other Creatures, as I have at large demonstrated in our Way to Health, Long Life and Happiness.

1. Bread and Water hath the first place of all Foods, and are the Foundation of dry moist nourishment, and of themselves being wisely prepared, make a good food of an opening, cleansing Nature and Operation, viz. Take Oatmeal and make it into Gruel, as we have Taught in our Monthly Observations of Health, then put bread into it; also take Water and good Wheat Flower [flour], and make it into a Pap, and put Bread into it, and season it with Salt; this and Bread with a Glass of Water, a Man may live very well, which a Friend of mine, of no mean Quality, has done for near two Years, eating neither Flesh, nor any of their Fruits, neither does he wear any Woolen Garments, but Linnen.

2. Bread and Butter, Bread and Cheese, being eaten alone, or with Sallad Herbs washed, without either Salt, Oil or Vinegar makes a most excellent Food, of a cleansing exhilarating Quality, easie of digestion; the frequent eating thereof, sweetens and generates good Blood, and fine Spirits, and prevents the generation of sower Humours, also keeps the body open; and all Herbs thus eaten, let the Food be what it will, is to be preferred before those that are eaten with Salt, Vinegar and Oil; especially for Women, and all Constitutions that are subject to generate sower Humours, and windy Diseases.

3. Bread and Butter eaten with our thin Gruel, wherein is only Salt to season it; the best way of eating it is to bite and Soop [dip], as you eat raw Milk and Bread; this is a most sweet and agreeable Food to the Stomach, of easie Concoction generates good Blood and causes it to Circulate freely, and is the most approved way of eating Water gruel with Butter.

4. Bread and Milk as it comes from the Cow, or raw, as they call it, is a most delicate Food, and Milk eaten thus is not only the best Food, but the most; the frequent eating thereof does sweeten the Blood, prevents sower Humours, carries Wind downward, and causes it to pass away freely without any trouble or molestation to Nature, but which the Stomach cannot so easily separate it, neither does it generate so fine Blood or Spirits; for this cause, if you boil Milk, and then set it to Cream, it will not separate, or afford more than a thick Skin; but remember that you do not eat your Milk before it be cold, not hot from the Cow as most incline to; the particular Reasons I have demonstrated in our *Good Housewife made a Doctor.*

5. Bread and Eggs, or Bread and raw Eggs, as they call them is an excellent Food, and it hath the first place of all Meats made of Eggs, being easier of Concoction, generates finer and better nourishment, it naturally cleanseth the passages, and the frequent eating of Bread and raw Eggs preserves the Lungs, the Bellows of Life, chears and warms the Stomach, and frees it from obstructions; but remember that you break both ends, and suck both the White and Yolk which contains the Spirits, and therefore they being eaten together, are both wholesomer than asunder and more agreeable to unto Nature; a little Custom will render them very pleasant and delightful to most, or all Constitutions.

6. Eggs, Parsley and Sorrel, mixed or stirred together, and Fried in a Pan with Butter and a little Salt, and when done, melt some Butter and Vinegar, and put on them, but you must not put too great a quantity of Herbs, for them it will render it more heavy and dull in Operation; this is a Noble and most delicious Dish and it affords a good nourishment, provided you eat not too much in quantity.

7. Eggs beaten together and Fried with Butter, and when done, melt some Butter and Vinegar and put over them is also a delightful and pleasant Dish, being much better and easier of Digestion, than the common way of Frying Eggs, as being lighter and more tender.

8. Eggs Poached, and some Parsley boiled and cut small, and mixed with some Butter and Vinegar melted, makes a very fine Dish and gives great satisfaction to the Stomach, supplying Nature with Nourishment to the highest degree, and is very grateful to the Palate.

9. Eggs boiled in their Shells, and Eggs Roasted, the last being the best, and eaten with Bread and Salt, or with Bread, Butter and Salt, is a good substantial Food; also Eggs broken and Butter'd over the Fire, is a good Food, being eaten without store of Bread.

10. Eggs being mixed with various sorts of Fruits, with Butter and Bread and made into Pies, is a sort of delicious Food, that a Man may give himself the Liberty to Eat now and then to great satisfaction, and not detriment to Nature, provided it not be too often.

11. Eggs Poached, and eaten with a Dish of boiled Spinnage [spinach] Buttered, is a good Food, and affords agreeable Nourishment, being eaten with plenty of good Bread.

12. Eggs with Flower and Water made into Pap on the Fire, as we have directed in the forementioned Book, *The Good Housewife made a Doctor*, is a Noble Food, affording a brave clean nourishment, being eaten either alone, or with Bread.

13. Raw Eggs, broke into our thin white Water Gruel, and Brewed together, with some Salt to season it, and then eaten with Bread, or Bread and Butter, makes a most exhilarating Food, being of a warming Quality, and unto the Stomach, generated good Blood, and fine brisk Spirits; this Gruel is very good for all young People and Women, for the frequent use of this, and others of our Spoon-Meats [liquid food], do naturally sweeten all the Humours, and prevents the generation of sower Juices, frees the passages from Windiness, and Griping pains.

14. Milk, Water and Flower, makes a brave substantial Pap or Food, this affords a strong Nourishment, and such as eat frequently of it, shall

not be subject neither to the gripes of the Stomach nor Bowels, and cuts off the generation of Wind in the bud, makes the Spirits brisk, the Body plump, fat, and of good Complexion, also it allays heat and drought, this being as friendly a Food to Nature as any Composition made by Fire with Milk.

15. One Egg broke into a Pint of good Ale, and Brewed well together, and eaten with Bread makes a brave Meal, and it hath a vigorous and quick operation in the Stomach; in the summer you may drink or eat it cold with Bread, but in the Winter warm it.

16. Take a Pint of good Ale, or good Beer, sweeten it with Sugar, then put it on the Fire, make it boiling hot, but not Boil, then take one or two Eggs, beat them with a little Water, then brew them well with your hot sweetened Ale or Beer; this is a Noble comforting sort of Food, or rather a rich Cordial, which does wonderfully replenish Nature with both dry and moist nourishment.

17. Rice and Water, boiled and buttered, is a friendly Food, and easie of Concoction, and affords a good nourishment.

18. Rice and Milk is also a noble Food affording a substantial nourishment, especially if you put Sugar in it, and remember, in what Spoon Meats soever you put butter, let no Sugar come and where you put Sugar let no Butter be.

19. An Egg or two beaten in a Pint of raw Milk, as they call it, either cold or warm according to the season of the year, is a noble substantial Food, affording a most excellent nourishment, the frequent eating thereof, prevents the generation of sower windy Humors (which are the original of many cruel Diseases, more especially in Women and Children), and gives all good healthy Complexion.

20. Milk made boiling hot, and then thickened with Eggs, is a brave substantial Food, of a friendly mild Nature and Operation, agreeable to most or all People.

21. There is also made of Milk, several other sorts of Foods, viz. Cheese-Cakes, Custards, White-Pots, all which are much of one Nature and Operation, they nourish much, and are substantial, but are not to be eaten too frequently.

22. Spinnage [spinach] boiled, or stewed, and buttered and eaten with Bread makes a brave cleansing Food, easie of Concoction, and generates good Blood, and sweetens the Humors, moves and opens Obstructions.

23. Spinnage, and the young buds of Colworts [cabbage] boiled in plenty of good Water, with a quick brisk Fire, and eaten only with Bread, Butter and Salt, is a fine pleasant delightful Food, affording good clean nourishment.

24. Spinnage, boiled with the sound tops of mint and Balm, seasoned with Salt and Butter, and eaten with Bread, makes a Noble Dish of a warming Quality, and gives great satisfaction to the Stomach, affording an excellent nourishment.

25. Spinnage, Endive, and young Parsley, boiled and eaten with Bread, Butter and Salt, is a brave friendly exhilarating Food, generating good Blood, and fine brisk Spirits, cleanseth the Passages, and loosens the Belly.

26. Boiled Cabbage, Collyflowers and Colworts, being eaten with Butter, Vinegar, Salt and Bread, the last of the three being the best, for they loosen up the Belly, purge by Urine, and are easie of Concoction, but remember that you boil them in plenty of good Water, with a quick Fire, and not too much, which is to be observed in all preparations of Herbs and Grains.

27. Asparagus, boiled and eaten with Bread, Butter and Salt, is a most delicious Food, it affords a clean nourishment, and is friendly to the Stomach, opens Obstructions, loosens the Belly, and powerfully purges by Urine.

28. Artichokes boiled, and eaten with Bread, Butter, and Salt, are an excellent Food, and generate a substantial nourishment; a Man may make a noble Meal of them.

29. Green Beans, boiled and eaten with Salt, Butter and Bread, is a most pleasant Food, they gently open the Belly, affording good nourishment, if you eat temperately of them, for they are an enticing Food. Let all People, subject to windy diseases, eat them sparingly.

30. French, or Kidney-Beans boiled in plenty of Water with a brisk Fire, and eaten with Bread, Butter and Salt, makes a brave delightful Dish of Food, of a cleansing opening nature and operation, they purge by Urine, and gently open the Belly, affording a good nourishment, provided they are eaten temperately; which is chiefly to be regarded in all green Foods.

31. Green Pease boiled, and seasoned with Salt and Butter, and eaten with Bread, makes a most pleasant Dish of Food; their nourishment is not strong, they are windy if not sparingly eaten.

32. Dry Pease being boiled in plenty of good soft Water, being seasoned with Salt and Butter, makes a substantial Dish of Food, and affords a strong nourishment, and is good for all strong labouring Men.

33. Boiled Turnips make a very good Dish of Food, being seasoned with Salt and Butter, and eaten with Bread, especially for all young People; they open and cleanse the Passages, and are easie of digestion, and may with safety be eaten plentifully; their colour declares their excellent Virtues.

34. Parsnips boiled in plenty of good Water, seasoned with Salt, Vinegar, Butter, and Mustard make a brave substantial hearty Dish of Food, and are friendly to most Constitutions.

35. Carrets boiled and seasoned with Salt and Butter, and eaten with good Bread, are a fine Dish of Food, very pleasant and wholsom, and are of easie Concoction; the deep red are best.

36. Roasted or boiled Potatoes eaten with Butter, Salt, and Vinegar, make a pleasant Dish of Food, very grateful to the Stomach, and are easie of digestion; now and then a Meal of them may do well.

37. Apple Dumplings eaten with Butter, or Butter and Sugar, hath the first place of most sorts of Puddings; they are easie of Concoction, and afford a friendly nourishment.

38. Plain Dumplings made very small, viz. with good Flower, Milk, Eggs, and a little Butter mixed or work'd up in them, and made thin like small Cakes, about as large as a Crown Piece, and put into boiling Water, which will be boiled in a little time; this is a noble substantial Food, very sweet and pleasant, of a warming nature, of an easie and friendly operation.

39. Plain Pudding made with Eggs, Flower, and Milk, well boiled and buttered, makes a firm Food, agreeable to the Stomach, being eaten temperately is both wholsom and healthy.

40. Boiled Dumplings made only with Flour, Milk or Water, with a little Ginger, which is the best Spice for Puddings, with Yeast or Barm, and when done buttered, is a very good wholsom Food, and of easie digestion; of this alone, a Man may now and then make a good Meal.

41. Boiled Pudding made with Flower, Milk and Eggs, and Raisons or Currans, and buttered, makes a pleasant Food, and a Man may now and then, give himself the liberty to make a Meal thereof without prejudice.

42. There are also several sorts of light Puddings made of Bread, and various sorts of ingredients, which are pleasant to the Palate, and not ungrateful to the Stomach, if sparingly eaten.

43. Rice Puddings both plain and made of Fruit, which for the most part are a pleasant sort of Food, easie of digestion, and may be freely eaten.

44. There are also several of Baked Puddings, which to most young People are delightful, they afford a good strong nourishment, and are best for such as Labour.

45. Apple Pies made with Fruit, that is neither too green or unripe, not too cold or far spent, are a very good Food, especially for young People; they afford a good nourishment, and are friendly to Nature.

46. Pear Pie being full, ripe, makes a fine, gentle, friendly Food of easie Concoction.

47. Rhadishes and Bread and Butter is a very good Food and a Man may now and then make a good Meal thereof; this affords a substantial nourishment far exceeding a Flesh Dinner.

48. Parsley and Bread and Butter, makes a noble and exhilarating Food, agreeable to Nature, nothing more friendly to the Stomach, breeds good Blood, and fine Spirits.

49. Sorrel and Bread and Butter, makes a brave, brisk Food, easie and quick of digestion, cleanseth the Stomach, and opens the Belly, and generates good Blood.

50. Balm and Bread and Butter, makes an excellent Food, of a chearing warming Quality; no sort of Food makes a better nourishment.

51. Sage and Bread and Butter, makes excellent Food, afford a good nourishment; its particular operation is, it warms the Stomach, and expels Wind.

52. Milk Pottage, viz. half Milk and half Water, mix it, and put it on our Fire, when boiling hot, then take it off the Fire, and brew it with some Oatmeal, ready tempered or mixed with a spoonful of cold Water or Milk, seasoned with Salt, and eaten with Bread, makes a very good substantial Food, affording a good nourishment, agreeable to the Stomach; but remember that it be made thin, and full half Water, otherwise it will be heavy on the Stomach; especially if it be for weakly Consumptive People.

53. There is also a brave sort of Food made of Wheat and Milk, called Furmity; some make it plain, and others add Fruit to it; the plain is the best, but they are both very good, affording a firm substantial nourishment, of a mild friendly operation; The frequent use of this is a grand enemy to the generation of sower windy Humours.

54. Boiled Wheat buttered is a noble Dish, and with this alone, a Man may make a better and more satisfactory Meal, than with Princely variety; it affords a sweet, friendly, and most agreeable nourishment, easie of concoction, and generates fine thin Blood.

55. Take good white Pease, boil them, when near done, add green Sage and Onions cut small, then season it with Salt and Butter; but in the Winter when green Sage is not good, then take that which is dried according to our Directions in the Way to Health, long Life and Happiness, which is to be preferred before green. This is a brave strong and substantial Pottage, very grateful to the Palate, and agreeable to the Stomach.

56. Directions to make several sorts of Herb Pottage, viz. take what quantity you please of good Water, make it boiling hot, then have our Herb or Herbs ready washed, not cut as the usual custom is; put them into your boiling hot Water, let your Vessel continue in the Fire till your Liquor begins to boil, then take it off the Fire, and let your Herbs remain in our boiling Liquor two or three Minutes; after which, take your Herbs out, then brew your hot Infusion with a little small Ground Oatmeal, which you must have ready, tempered with a Spoonful or two of cold Water, adding Salt and Butter to it, which ought to be brewed with your Oatmeal. This Pottage or Gruel, you may eat with Bread or without, as you find most agreeable to your Stomach; all Herb Pottages made after this method, are far more commendable, for all good purposes, than that made the common and usual way, for the hot Liquor, in a moments time, draws forth all the fine, spirituous Virtues, and strength of the Malt; for in most, or all Infusions, the fine spirituous qualities separate, and do first give themselves into any proper Minstruum, or Liquor.

57. Smallage [wild celery] makes a Pottage or Gruel of a cleansing quality, it purifies the Blood, opens Obstructions of the Liver and Spleen; this Pottage alone eaten twice a day, is an effectual Remedy against all Consumptive Humours.

58. Sellary [celery] does also make a brave Physical Pottage, it warms and comforts the Spirits, affords a good nourishment, and is an admirable Remedy against Windy Humours.

59. Leek Pottage is not only good Food, but is also profitable against short windedness, and other Obstructions or the Uriters, and is good against short windedness, and other Obstructions of the Breast, and affords a good clean nourishment.

60. Onion Pottage; this eaten with good Bread, Butter, and Salt, makes a brave Meal of itself; it is also good against difficult breathing.

61. Garlick Pottage is chiefly good for full Bodied Corpulent Men, and such as are troubled with Coughs, the Stone and Gravel.

62. Parsley Pottage warms the Stomach, chears the Spirits, and is very agreeable to the Stomach, being eaten with Bread, Butter, and Salt; a Man may make a very good Meal thereof.

63. Mint makes a noble exhilarating Pottage, the frequent eating thereof, does not only prevent windy Humours in the Passages, but it mightily strengthens the Retentive Faculty of the Stomach.

64. Balm makes a Pottage of a warming comforting quality, and is a gallant Food, affording excellent nourishment; this alone makes a noble Meal, to the highest satisfaction of the Stomach.

65. Water-Cresses made into Pottage being eaten with Bread, Butter, and Salt, is not only a good Food, but the frequent use thereof cleanseth the Blood, and prevents Fumes and Vapours from flying into the Crown.

66. Sweet Charwell makes and excellent Pottage, being eaten with Bread, Butter, and Salt, is not only a brave Food, but it warms cold Stomachs, and is a friend to the Lungs.

67. Take Currans, boil them in your Water, when almost done, mix a little small Oatmeal with two Spoonfuls of cold Water, stir it in, and let it boil a little; when done, season it with Salt, adding Sugar with it; This eaten with Bread makes a good Meal. You may add Butter as most good Housewives do, but I must tell them that it makes it heavy on the Stomach, and apt to send Fumes into the Head.

68. Boil your Raisins in Water, as is mentioned before of Currans, when almost done, then stir your tempered Oatmeal in and let it boil a small time, when done, add Salt, Sugar, and Bread; you may add Butter, especially if the Eaters thereof be strong working People; this Pottage affords much nourishment, and a Man may sometimes make a very good Meal of this alone.

69. Take Raisins, Currans and a few Pruens and boil them in good Water, when near done thicken it with white Bread, adding Spice, Sugar, Butter, and Salt; this is a rich Pottage, affording a great nourishment, and therefore it must be eaten the more sparingly.

70. A piece of good Bread, and a Pint of good Ale or Beer, makes a very gallant Meal, it warms the Stomach, is easie of digestion, generates good Blood, and it has a quick and pleasant Operation.

71. Bread and half a Pint of good Canary Wine, a Man may make a noble and most delightful Meal, even to the highest satisfaction of Nature.

72. Bread and a Pint of Good Cyder, do also make a good Meal, it breeds good nourishment and makes a Man full of Life and Spirit.

73. Bread and half a pint of Cherry Wine, Gooseberry Wine or Currans Wine, with this alone a Man may make a brave Dinner, is affords a noble brisk Spirit and nourishment.

74. Flummery [oatmeal porridge] is an ancient Food the Britains used to eat, and the use of it is still continued amongst the Welsh; the Britains, and those that now eat this sort of Gruel, had, and have various ways of eating it, viz. to mix Ale with it, and so eat it with Bread, others Milk, Cream and the like; which mixtures do very well. This Gruel I recommend to all weak Stomach'd People, and especially to such whose Breasts and Passages are furred, and obstructed by sweet tough, and phlegmy Matter, it being an excellent remedy against all such infirmities.

75. Bonniclabber is a sort of Milk Meat, and though last spoken of, deserves the first place for its excellent Virtues; Boniclabber is nothing else but Milk that has stood till it is sower, and become of a thick slippery substance; this is an excellent Food being eaten with good Bread in hot Seasons, especially for Consumptive People, and such as are trouble with any kind of stoppages of the Breast, it naturally opens the Passages, its easie of concoction, and helps digest all hard or sweeter Foods, it also cools and cleanseth the whole Body, and renders it brisk and lively, quencheth Thirst to admiration: and with this, or any of the forementioned Dishes of Food, any Person may make a hearty Meal thereof with great satisfaction.

Resources

In this section you will find helpful links to the official web site for *The Benjamin Franklin Diet* as well as suppliers that sell whole grains, grain mills, spices, cheese-making supplies, and similar.

Atlantic Spice
2 Shore Rd.
North Truro, MA 02652
Phone: 800-316-7965
Website: www.atlanticspice.com

Wholesale suppliers of whole and ground spices, sea salt, extracts, flavorings, spice jars, mortar and pestles, tea bags, tea balls, and more. Great prices. Minimum order $30.

Homebrewer's Outpost
801 S. Milton Rd, Suite #2
Flagstaff, AZ 86001
Phone: 928-774-2499 or 800-450-9535
Website: www.homebrewers.com

Suppliers of homemade soda flavors, extracts, and soda-making kits to brew root beer, ginger beer, and other homemade sodas. Also carry empty root beer bottles, and supplies for making beer and wine.

Pleasant Hill Grain
210 South 1st Street
P.O. Box 7
Hampton, Nebraska 68843-0007
Phone: 402-725-3835 or 800-321-1073
Website: www.pleasanthillgrain.com

Suppliers of electric and hand-operated grain mills, whole organic grains, including wheat, rye, oats, corn, and many more. Also carry baking pans, butter crocks, and breadmaking supplies. Family-operated business with great prices, great service, and fast shipping.

www.thebenjaminfranklindiet.com

Visit the official web site of The Benjamin Franklin Diet *for more of Kelly Wright's Ben-friendly recipes, health and fitness articles, dieting tips and the latest news.*

References

Parts One and Two

Aceto, C., Stoppani, J. "Twelve Laws of Fat-Burning." Muscleandfitness.com

Barr, SL. "Reduce the Size of Your Tummy, Say Diet Experts, and You'll Eat Less and Drop Unwanted Pounds." *Good Housekeeping*, July 1, 1997.

Davis, A. *Let's Eat Right to Keep Fit.* New York, NY: Harcourt Brace Jovanovich, Inc, 1970.

d'Elgin, T. *What Should I Eat? A Complete Guide to the New Food Pyramid.* New York, NY: Ballantine Books, 2005.

"Diet in the Roman Army." http://www.museumreplicas.com/t-romandiet.aspx

Franklin, B. *Poor Richard.* Philadelphia, PA: B. Franklin & D. Hall, 1733. (The Franklin Collection, Yale University Library)

Franklin, B. *Poor Richard Improved.* Philadelphia, PA: B. Franklin & D. Hall, 1756. (The Franklin Collection, Yale University Library)

Franklin, B. *A Dissertation on Liberty and Necessity, Pleasure and Pain.* London, England, 1725. (The Franklin Collection, Yale University Library)

Franklin, B. *Letter to Deborah Franklin.* 1756.

Franklin, B. *Poor Richard Improved.* Philadelphia, PA: B. Franklin & D. Hall, 1765. (The Franklin Collection, Yale University Library)

Franklin, B. *Letter as "Homespun"* in: *The Gazetteer and New Daily Advertiser.* January 2, 1766.

Franklin, B. *Notes on a Week's Diet and Poor Health.* 1769. (The Franklin Collection, Yale University Library)

Franklin, B. *Letter to William Franklin*. 1772.

Franklin, B. *Poor Richard Improved*. Philadelphia, PA: B. Franklin & D. Hall, 1772. (The Franklin Collection, Yale University Library)

Franklin, B. *Letter on Maize*. 1785.

Franklin, B. *Letter to Catherine Shipley*. 1786.

Franklin, B. "The Morals of Chess." *The Columbian Magazine*, The American Philosophical Society. December, 1786.

Franklin, B. *Autobiography*. 1790.

Franklin, B. *Autobiography*. Introduction by Daniel Aaron. New York, NY: Vintage Books, 1987.

Hawke, DF. *Everyday Life in Early America*. New York, NY: Harper & Row, 1988.

How to Use Fruits and Vegetables to Help Manage Your Weight, Centers for Disease Control and Prevention, http://www.cdc.gov/healthyweight/healthy_eating/fruits_vegetables.html

Isaacson, W. *Benjamin Franklin, An American Life*. New York, NY: Simon & Schuster, 2003.

Lappé, FM. *Diet for a Small Planet*. New York, NY: Ballantine Books, 1971.

Mellen, P., et al. "Health Benefits of Whole Grains Confirmed." *Science Daily*, May 10, 2007.

Morrison, M. *Doctor Morrison's Miracle Guide to Pain-Free Health and Longevity*. West Nyack, NY: Parker Publishing Company, Inc., 1977.

National Health and Nutrition Examination Survey 1999–2000. http://www.faqs.org/nutrition/Met-Obe/National-Health-and-Nutrition-Examination-Survey-NHANES.html. National Center for Health Statistics (NCHS)

O'Brien, JE. *Herbal Cures for Common Ailments*. New York, NY: Globe Digest Series, 2000.

Okot, HS. "How to Shrink Your Tummy." Monitor Online, March 27, 2008.

On Independence Day, Nutritionists Cast a Cold Eye on Eating Habits of Colonial America, June 24, 2000. http://www.charitywire.com/charity10/00210.html

Prevention Magazine Editorial Staff. *Natural Weight Loss*. Emmaus, PA: Rodale Press, 1985.

"A Quick Biography of Benjamin Franklin." *The Electric Ben Franklin.* http://www.ushistory.org/franklin/info/index.htm

"The 20 Health Benefits of Real Butter." *Body Ecology.* http://www.bodyecology.com/07/07/05/benefits_of_real_butter.php

Tunis, E. *Colonial Living.* Cleveland, OH: World Publishing Company, 1957.

What Is a GMO? GMO Basics, Institute for Responsible Technology. www.responsibletechnology.org

http://www.quakeroats.com/quaker-for-health-care-professionals.aspx

Part Three—Cookbooks

Alley, L. *Lost Arts.* Berkeley, CA: Ten Speed Press, 1995.

Davis, A. *Let's Cook It Right.* New York, NY: Harcourt Brace Jovanovich, Inc, 1947.

The Edinburgh Book of Plain Cookery Recipes - Revised and Enlarged Edition. London, England: Thomas Nelson and Sons, Ltd, 1932.

Elverson, VT, McLanahan, MA. *A Cooking Legacy.* New York, NY: Walker and Company, 1975.

Franklin, B. *Letter to James Bowden.* 1763.

Franklin, B. *Letter to David LeRoy.* 1784.

Franklin, B. *Letter Recipe for Making Bread of Maize and Wheat Flour.* February 5, 1784 (The Franklin Collection, Yale University Library)

Keller, A. *Grandma's Cooking.* New York, NY: Prentice Hall, Inc, 1955.

The Old Farmer's Almanac Colonial Cookbook. Dublin, NH: Yankee Publishing Inc., 1976.

Reader's Digest Editorial Staff. *Back to Basics: How to Learn and Enjoy Traditional American Skills,* Second Edition. Pleasantville, NY: Reader's Digest Books, 1996.

Reno, K. *Perfumes, Potions & Fanciful Formulas.* Monrovia, CA: Victorian Essence Press, 1998.

Simmons, A. *American Cookery: Or, The Art of Dressing Viands, Fish, Poultry and Vegetables, and the Best Modes of Making Pastes, Puffs, Pies, Tarts, Puddings, Custards, and Preserves.* Hartford, CT: Hudson and Goodwin, Printers, 1796. (This first American cookbook was originally printed for its author. There have been many reprints over time.)

Tighe, E., Editor. *Woman's Day Encyclopedia of Cookery, Volume 9, Pennsylvania Dutch Cookery.* New York, NY: Fawcett Publications, 1966.

Tryon, T. *Wisdom's Dictates: or Aphorism's and Rules, Physical, Moral and Divine; For By Preserving the Health of the Body and the Peace of the Mind, fit to be regarded and practiced by all that would enjoy the Blessings of the present and future World; A Bill of Fare Of Seventy five Noble Dishes of Excellent Food, far exceeding those made of Fish and Flesh, which Banquet I present to the Sons of Wisdom, or such as shall decline that depraved Custom of Eating Flesh and Blood.* London, England: Thomas Salisbury, 1691.

Walker, Bev. *The Amazing All-Purpose Pine Needle Tea,* February 25, 2011, www.davesgarden.com/guides/articles/view/3126

Westland, P. *Spices, How to Select, Grow, Preserve and Cook With Spices.* New York, NY: Exeter Books, 1985.

Women's Institute of Domestic Arts and Sciences, Inc. *Women's Institute Library of Cookery Volume One: Essentials of Cookery; Cereals; Breads; Hot Breads.* Scranton, PA: Women's Institute of Domestic Arts and Sciences, 1917.

Index

About the Author

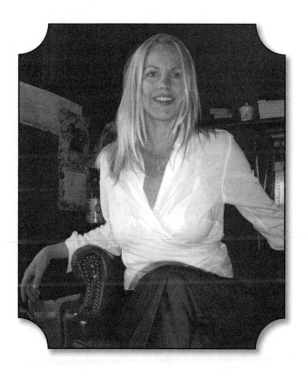

Kelly Wright has had fourteen books published across a wide spectrum of topics. Their many genres range from non-fiction titles on health, beauty, careers, and small business, to a series of horror novels and romantic fantasy. Kelly resides in Big Bear Lake, California, where, in addition to writing, she enjoys skiing, fishing, and playing in the great outdoors with her husband, Tommy, and baby daughter, Ruby Lee.

Notes

Notes

Notes

Notes